Meat, Muscle and Mind

The Carnivore Way of Eating Naturally

James Barbour

Dedication

This book is dedicated to the loving memory of my mother, Marcille Barbour. Marcille was a vibrant woman who had a smile for everyone and elevated the mood in every room. Marcille raised 5 children, of which I am the oldest.

Being the oldest, it was incumbent on me to "Set the example" for the other four. This was my mother's way of keeping me in line and out of trouble. I think she learned the psychology of this from the Catholic Church.

Her handwriting was immaculate, so there was no way to forge any "notes from home" when I got into trouble. My mother was very artsy and crafty. She had a knack for creating beautiful objects out of simple items. She designed and decorated our entire house. I remember when she converted our basement into a family room, she came up with a plan to decorate using an old sword that her father had given her. She designed a family crest using a plaster mold, painted it with skill, and crisscrossed the swords behind it.

Needless to say, she didn't like it and wanted to start over with a new idea. The new concept consisted of a 2' x 2' copper sheet, black spray paint, and a wooden dowel. I watched in amazement as she sprayed one side completely black and then used the dowel to press a design into the copper to gradually create a bust of a medieval "knight" on the unpainted side of the copper. The amazing part is that it was the backside of the piece, so everything she was designing was in reverse from a normal perspective. Once the details of the face were etched into the copper, she used steel wool to lightly remove some black paint from the front of the piece, revealing the gleaming copper design. The result was amazing!

One year, she decided to enter the town door decorating contest for the Christmas Holiday. This consisted of chicken wire, four 8' pieces of 1"x3" lumber, and a quick trip to the woods to "borrow" some evergreen branches. My mother proceeded to construct a full-sized Christmas tree, 3 dimensional, facing the road, but flat on the backside to easily attach to the front door. Once it was up and fully decorated, there was no doubt that this door would be hard to beat! A few days later, my mother and the new tree door are in the local paper, "The Cheshire Herald," and are the proud winners of the Door Decorating Contest!

One day, I came home from High School to find my mother crying. This was a very rare event. She didn't want to discuss the issue, but when I pressed it, she revealed that she had been diagnosed with breast cancer. The always happy and cheerful mother that I had known was now quiet, sad, and tearful.

What came next was many rounds of chemo, hair loss, and endless waiting for the phone to ring with the news of how the treatments were going. Luckily, the treatments worked well, and her cancer retreated. The checkups and follow-up calls gradually became further apart over time, and things returned to normal. Laughter and fun came back into our world for many years.

It was 18 years later that I got a phone call from my mother. Her cancer had metastasized in her body in a few places. Since so much time had passed and the advancement in medicine was great, I felt that she would beat this once again. Each medication they tried had little to no impact on the cancer, and it continued spreading. On August 3rd, 2011, we lost my mother to cancer at the age of 67.

My mother did things by the book. She did not smoke, rarely had a drink, and was in good shape. My reflection on her cancer diagnosis was that she was unfortunate to have come down with the disease that cut her life short. This made me question, "Did the Standard American Diet have anything to do with her cancer?"

Acknowledgment

I was searching on YouTube for healthier ways to address my type 2 diabetes when I stumbled across the Carnivore Diet and the following authorities that made me think hard about our food habits and the ingredients we put into our bodies.

I am not a medical professional or a doctor; I am a layperson who simply wants to understand the impacts of the food we put into our bodies. My research journey has opened my eyes to so much information that I felt compelled to put this book together. I hope to boil down the data in a way that makes sense to the average person looking to eat for health rather than for entertainment.

The content provided, including any discussions related to health, diet, or medical conditions, is for informational purposes only and is not intended to be a substitute for professional medical advice, diagnosis, or treatment. Each individual has a unique body which may react differently to food ingredients. Always seek the advice of your physician or other qualified health provider with any questions you may have regarding a medical condition or dietary change. My personal experiences or insights should not be interpreted as medical advice.

When I first began my journey, the following authorities shaped my thoughts on "The Carnivore Diet," and all have large audiences on YouTube:

Stella, "The Steak and Butter Gal" was my introduction to the Carnivore way of eating. She has been a carnivore for 5 years with amazing results. Prior to the Carnivore diet, she had several years of the Vegan lifestyle but experienced several issues such as acne, bloating, and fatigue, which were all "self-cured" without medication due to the Carnivore diet. Today, Bella has created the online community "The Steak and Butter Gang," comprising like-minded people looking for a healthier lifestyle backed by a panel of experts. I found Stella to be an amazing teacher with proven results on this diet. Her YouTube channel has great content, with over 40 million views as of September 2024.

Dr. Ken Berry coined the Phrase "Proper Human Diet (PHD)," and it makes so much sense. In his own words, he used to be a "Fat, pre-diabetic, miserable, family physician" before he realized he was mistaught and misled about food. Humans used to be hunters and gatherers for sources of nutrition that were low in carbohydrates and not factory-made, with no extra steps added to "make" the food and no added sugars to taste better.

Jordan Peterson—I knew that Jordan Peterson was a Canadian psychologist, professor, and well-known author with very intelligent views on psychology, philosophy, and cultural issues. What I didn't know was that this smart man had adopted the Carnivore Diet. This gave me reassurance that the diet may not be a "fad" and have some real benefits. Later, I discovered that his daughter, Mikhaila Peterson, is known for her work as a health and wellness advocate. She has gained attention for her views on diet, particularly her promotion of the carnivore diet, which emphasizes animal products. Mikhaila has also shared her personal health journey, including her struggles with autoimmune issues. She runs a podcast where she discusses various topics related to health, wellness, and culture, often featuring guests from diverse fields.

Dr. Eric Berg is a chiropractor and health educator known for his focus on ketogenic diets, intermittent fasting, and overall wellness. He has a strong online presence, particularly on platforms like YouTube, where he shares educational videos on topics related to nutrition, weight loss, and health improvement. Dr. Berg emphasizes the importance of understanding the body's metabolic processes and offers advice on dietary strategies for achieving optimal health. His approach often includes practical tips for lifestyle changes aimed at improving well-being.

Dr. Anthony Chaffee is a medical doctor and advocate for the carnivore diet, which emphasizes a diet primarily consisting of animal products. He shares insights on nutrition, health, and wellness, often discussing the potential benefits of a meat-based diet for various health conditions. Dr. Chaffee has a presence on social media and podcasts, where he explores topics related to dietary choices, lifestyle, and overall health. His views are part of a broader conversation about nutrition and its impact on well-being.

Dr. Eric Westman is a physician and a prominent advocate of the ketogenic diet, particularly in the context of treating obesity and type 2 diabetes. He is the co-founder of the 'Duke Lifestyle Medicine Clinic' and has researched low-carbohydrate diets and their effects on health. Dr. Westman has authored books and numerous studies focusing on how dietary interventions can lead to significant health improvements. He often speaks at conferences and contributes to discussions about nutrition and metabolic health, promoting the benefits of low-carb and ketogenic diets for weight management and overall well-being.

Lastly, HomesteadHow is about a family of six who left the city to live and grow on a 20-acre farm. Kerry is a Carnivore who created a documentary, 'Healing Humanity- The Power of a Proper Human Diet,' which explored the effect of a proper human diet on various health-related issues.

About the Author

Born in the late '60s, James missed out on the adventures of Woodstock but always loved the classic rock of the 60s and 70s born from that era.

Raised in New England, James was always close to nature and enjoyed hiking in the mountains and fishing in the rivers and ocean of Long Island Sound from the shores of Connecticut. To this day, James loves camping in Nature, moving around the country in his Sprinter Van RV.

Growing up, James enjoyed bike riding and playing sports with the neighborhood kids – nerf football, wiffleball, little league baseball, bowling, and even a short stint on the high school golf team. He was thin growing up and never tried out for the football team. He chalked that up to being smart and not wanting to get injured!

James grew up eating the normal American Diet foods and never thought about the contents or ramifications of the food he consumed. Cereal is for breakfast, hot dogs or cold cuts are for lunch, and chocolate milk and ring dings are available at school. Dinners were typically some sort of meat and potatoes and a vegetable [canned] and the occasional dessert of brownies, cake, or ice cream. Friday nights usually consisted of a big pasta dish or Pizza [his favorite].

James went to college at Lehigh University in Bethlehem, PA, in the late 1980s and eventually became an entrepreneur. He started an IT Consulting company near Baltimore, Maryland. All this time, eating the Standard American diet without regard or regrets.

And yet, for the last 8 years, James Barbour had been trying to understand the events that led to his diagnosis of being prediabetic. All outward signs appeared to be normal; he had a slender build, was a non-smoker, was relatively active in outdoor activities, and happily ate a wide variety of foods.

But little did he know, he had slowly contaminated his body for nearly 5 decades!

Preface

I never thought I'd say this, but the day I bit into a juicy steak after years of being a "health-conscious" eater was the day my life changed forever. It was a moment that would have sent my old self into a fit. I mean, as an avid advocate for the healthy 'American Diet,' how could I just turn a blind eye to all that had brought me there? However, the fact of the matter was that I was pre-diabetic. Despite my diligence and efforts to be a healthy eater, my body was turning on me, and I felt lost at sea.

It was one of those moments when desperation made me ask myself the most radical question: What if everything I thought I knew about nutrition was wrong? It was at this point in my journey that I stumbled upon the carnivore diet on the internet. It was ludicrous, and yet it was hard to put down. Did the entire meat industry get a bad rap? Here's the story of my journey from a plate of hamburgers to a sizzling ribeye, full of skepticism and humor.

However, this book is more than just my story; it's a challenge to the norms we've come to accept about food. Together, we'll explore the myth of the "healthy" diet and examine how the foods we've been told are good for us might be causing harm. You will learn from real athletes like Adam Peaty, who returned from veganism to eating animal-based proteins to meet his demanding training needs. You will learn how the science of our food choices impacts our lives and how even your kale smoothie is not as innocent as it appears.

So, buckle up, dear reader. Let's explore what if the road to perfect health was made of…bacon. Well, come and discover a world where the assumptions about food that have plagued our minds for far too long are turned upside-down. This is not simply a diet—it's a revolution. It's the trip of redemption with one bite at a time.

Contents

Introduction: The Day I Ate My Words (And a Lot of Meat)

Would you believe me if I told you that eating meat can increase the risk of certain cancers? And would you believe me if I told you eating too many vegetables can lead to gut issues and kidney problems?

Both of these claims are under-researched and do not have significant evidence backing them up, yet we are more inclined to believe the first statement to be true. Why is that you might ask. It's because we are trained to think that meat – especially red meat – is bad for our health. But how much truth is there in that? Let's discuss this through my example. I learned firsthand how deeply ingrained our misconceptions about food can be when I discovered my pre-diabetes diagnosis—despite living what I thought was a healthy lifestyle.

I was a 'healthy' 50-year-old man. I showed no symptoms of any illness, I wasn't overweight, and I was not taking any medication. I cared for my health well and had the same diet as an average American. So, imagine my surprise when I found out I was pre-diabetic during a routine physical test.

To say I was shocked would be an understatement. No one in my family – that I knew of – had diabetes. So, it couldn't have been genetic. I took my walks and did my exercises, which didn't make sense either. The only thing that stood out to me was my diet. But I had a balanced diet; I ate my greens and took my vitamins, and yet still, I was at risk of diabetes.

The doctor recommended some preventative meds. But medications often come with side effects, and they don't necessarily address the underlying issue—they just mask it. And then, you become dependent on these meds to mask the underlying cause of the problem. I am not one to accept being on medications for the rest of my life, which is why I decided to take matters into my own hands and get to the bottom of this issue.

In a moment of desperation, I thought of a crazy idea: "What if everything I thought I knew about nutrition was wrong?" That led to a late-night internet trip down the proverbial "rabbit hole." I looked up all the different types of diets and their potential for getting rid of pre-diabetes. Was I ready physically and emotionally to challenge the dietary norms of the Standard American Diet that I had faithfully followed for 50-plus years?

At first, I took baby steps. I completely stopped drinking soda and eliminated sugar from my coffee. This was a big difference in taste, but I quickly got used to coffee without sugar, and it was not bad! I walked a little bit more regularly and increased the distance gradually. I significantly reduced *refined* and *processed* foods. Although my blood sugar results improved, it was not to the extent that I had hoped.

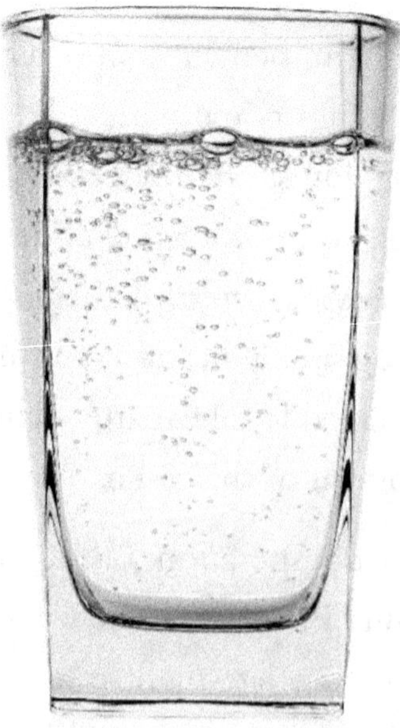

I needed to do more, so I started reading labels. I was shocked at the amount of sugar in just about everything in the grocery store. I saw so many ingredients that were not natural sounding and many that were meant to increase the shelf life of this processed food. It was then that I discovered the carnivore diet.

In the beginning, it sounded absurd to me. What do you mean that I should only eat meat and NO vegetables? What of all the teachers, doctors, and moms who told me to eat my greens? How else would I get my micro-nutrients? As children, we were advised to eat 2-3 cups of vegetables daily. Turned out it was all a marketing plan that became the basis of the "healthy" eating recommendations of the United States Department of Agriculture (USDA) – 4 Food Groups. This eventually led to the "Food Pyramid" and its subsequent variations.

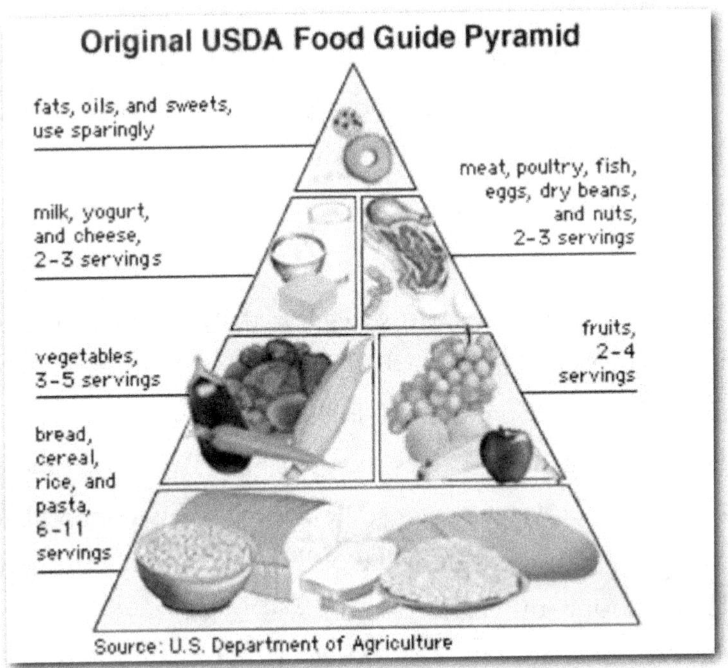

Despite my reservations, I decided to give the carnivore diet a chance out of desperation. I started the Carnivore Diet as a test 90 days ago and have continued it for 1 year now. I never thought I'd say this, but the day

I bit into a juicy steak after years of being a 'health-conscious' individual, my life changed forever.

I had consulted the biggest meat-loving friend I could think of and went out to dinner with him. I asked him to order for me, and here I was, staring at a plate of ribeye like it was about to grow legs and run away. I'd never seen that much meat on a plate. The steak he ordered for me was enormous. It glistened with juices that seemed to mock me, daring me to take a bite. My usual meals were a colorful medley of greens and grains that made people say, "You must be very healthy." But tonight, I was crossing into uncharted territory—a full-blown carnivore's paradise.

I could almost hear my vegetarian friends gasping in horror. In my mind, they had already formed an intervention group chat. I knew their messages would ping with urgency: "Is this a cry for help?" one might ask, while another would suggest, "Maybe it's just a phase, like that time he thought he could pull off a mullet." I thought deeply about my vegan friend's will to eat a special diet and the challenges they must have faced. If they could do it, then so could I!

As I picked up my knife and fork, I felt a pang of guilt. But not just for the cow but for betraying the unspoken health code. I had spent years perfecting the art of the balanced meal. I was about to demolish a ribeye that could feed a small village. How could eating red meat with fat be a healthy move? The pressure was real.

The first bite was a revelation. Juicy, rich, and flavorful—it was better than anything I had ever tasted. I half-expected a choir of angels to start singing. But then, I wondered when the meat sweats would kick in. It never happened to me, but I have heard it impacted some people.

Once an object of terror, the steak now felt like a challenge I was determined to conquer. By the time I had finished, I was both victorious and defeated. I was left questioning my life choices once the plate was clean.

At first, I didn't notice any change, but over time, problems I didn't think I had improved. Even before I got my blood test done, I knew this diet was working. The stubborn belly fat was slowly vanishing, I was sleeping better, my skin improved, and all of these changes were visible from the first month.

A few weeks after starting the carnivore diet, I noticed some unexpected physical and mental shifts. One of the most notable changes had been the surge in energy levels - I found myself feeling more alert and ready to tackle the day.

With more energy, I was surprised to also feel a boost in mental clarity. Additionally, I observed a gradual disappearance of chronic symptoms that I had been dealing with before. It was a fascinating and somewhat unexpected transformation. But it was quite a journey.

The turning point came during a follow-up doctor's appointment just 90 days after starting the carnivore lifestyle. I had braced myself for the bad news. I was expecting the doctor to tell me my cholesterol levels had skyrocketed or that I had developed some rare meat-related ailment. Instead, the results were astonishing. My health markers had improved dramatically. Blood sugar panels? Perfect. Cholesterol? Better than ever. However, my blood pressure was still a bit higher than ideal. I have been getting high readings for blood pressure over the last few years and got anxious each time I had to take the test, which was another reason I investigated the carnivore diet.

I read that one of the benefits of a carnivore diet was removing inflammation from the body. Which, over time, lowers blood pressure. That was a great goal for me.

My physician, who had delivered the bad – pre-diabetic – news to me a few months ago, was left in disbelief. "I don't know what you're doing, but keep doing it," she said, shaking her head in wonder. She followed that up with, "If your next blood pressure reading is high, we will need to address that."

This unexpected validation gave me the confidence to continue my carnivorous journey despite the social awkwardness and raised eyebrows. It took me 50 years to develop these symptoms, so I figured that my blood pressure would take some time to adjust as well.

I started to question the long-held beliefs I had about vegetable consumption and the American Standard diet of processed foods. Could a powerful lobby for the processed food industry and Big Pharma have misled us? I mean, they were eager to sell drugs to manage the health issues caused by poor diet, so it made sense. The deeper I dove into the research, the more I realized how skewed and biased much of the information was. This realization fueled my determination to explore the carnivore diet further.

Do not get me wrong, I have always believed that vegetables were good for you since they were natural and grown from the ground. The thing I started questioning about was "How" the vegetables were raised and delivered to the grocery store. A little research showed that mass-scale farming strips the land of nutrients and breeds various insects, critters, mold, and mildew.

To combat this, the recommended path is fertilizer and pesticides. I began to wonder how much of that actually gets into our bodies. Another thing I began to question was how a loaf of white bread could maintain its freshness for over 2 weeks when homemade bread starts to mold in 3 days.

When you look up the disadvantages of eating a vegetarian diet on the internet, you get results like *Side Effects of Eating Vegetables* and *what happens when you overconsume vegetables*. On the other hand, if you look up the disadvantages of eating a carnivore diet, you will find the *disadvantages of eating meat. A meat-only diet is not the answer,* and my personal favorite: *The risks of a carnivore diet.*

Do you see the difference between the choice of words for each topic? For a veg-only diet, they use terms like 'side effects' and 'overconsumption,' but for its carnivore counterpart, more anxiety-inducing words like 'risks' are used. This association of harsher words for a carnivore diet in social spaces makes it difficult for us to try it out.

We have all fallen for this unfavorable language and believe it to be true. This subtle language has created an inherent fear of meat in our minds. The second we enter the red meat section of a grocery store, a big red CHOLESTROL flag waves in our minds. I found myself in a similar situation quite a few times. I was at the local grocery store one Sunday and was doing my weekly shopping. I headed straight for the meat counter and skipped the produce section where I had spent so many years meticulously selecting the freshest vegetables.

As I loaded my cart with steaks, bacon, eggs, hamburgers, chicken breasts, and pork chops, I could feel the eyes of fellow shoppers boring into my back.

At the checkout, an older woman behind me analyzed my purchases. "That's a lot of meat. Are you having a BBQ?" she commented, her tone conversational.

"Nope," I replied cheerfully, "I'm on an all-animal product diet."

Her eyes widened in shock. "You know that's not healthy, right? Red meat is terrible for your heart."

I took a deep breath, resisting the urge to roll my eyes. "Actually, I have done a lot of research, and it's working well for me. My health has improved significantly, and I am no longer pre-diabetic. Plus, I feel great."

She huffed, clearly unimpressed. "Well, I hope you know what you're doing," she muttered, turning her attention to the organic carrots and kale in her cart.

I couldn't help but chuckle as I left the store. It was a small encounter, but it perfectly encapsulated the judgment and misconceptions I faced daily. Yet, there were moments of genuine curiosity and interest for every disapproving glance.

It reminded me that change is often met with resistance, especially in something as personal as diet. But with each conversation and explanation, I was helping to challenge the narrative and open minds. It was one grocery store showdown at a time. Switching to an all-animal product diet pushed me into a series of awkward social situations. Dinner parties became a minefield. I was used to navigating the buffet table with the ease of a seasoned 'health enthusiast,' but now I found myself in uncharted territory.

"A salad for you?" hosts would ask. "Actually, I'll take the steak," I'd reply, causing a few raised eyebrows and a lot of surprised gasps.

Some restaurants were experienced with the carnivore diet, and that gave me some comfort. It was fairly easy to order a steak, but you would get some eyes when you declined the salad, the bread, the veggies, and the baked potato. I did enjoy ordering a juicy burger. However, "2 burgers with cheese and bacon, no veggies, no bun" raises some eyebrows. What truly puzzled them was the polite decline to say, "Would you like fries with that?"

I remember the first time I told my friends about my new carnivore diet. We gathered at my friend's place and sat around the table. I hesitated, but finally, I cleared my throat.

"Um, I have a bit of a confession," I began, "I am a carnivore now." It felt like I was coming out.

"What do you mean?" one asked.

"It means I only eat meat and animal products," I explained.

"Are you serious?" she asked, scandalized.

"Dead serious," I replied, trying to muster a confident smile. Then began a flurry of questions and concerns. "Isn't that unhealthy?" "What about your cholesterol?" "Have you lost your mind?"

As the interrogation continued, I couldn't help but feel like a defendant in a dietary trial. But then, one of my fitness enthusiast friends chimed in. "Actually, I've heard about the benefits of a high-protein diet," he said. "It's controversial, but some people swear by it."

His words were a small victory. There was finally a crack in the wall of skepticism. By the night's end, curiosity replaced judgment, and my friends asked for updates on my health journey.

My family always supported my decisions but couldn't understand my sudden dietary shift. "But you loved my veggie lasagna!" my mom exclaimed as if my new carnivorous ways were a personal insult to her cooking.

Thanks to one-sided marketing and outdated health recommendations, eating meat has always gotten a bad rap. Red meat is deemed the big, bad villain. It is blamed for everything from bad cholesterol to heart disease. Knowing what I know now, the food pyramid – with its heavy emphasis on grains and minimal meat – seems more like a guideline for disaster than a path to health.

Determined to uncover the truth, I decided to dive deeper into the science behind the carnivore diet. I read studies, listened to experts, and analyzed data. What I found was astonishing. Not only were there numerous health benefits to an all-meat diet, but many people had experienced significant improvements in their well-being, just like I had.

If I could find healing through natural animal products, how many others out there were suffering needlessly? This is why I felt compelled to share my journey with others.

We are about to embark on a journey to challenge everything you thought you knew about food. And trust me, it's going to be one hell of a ride. With these words, I invite you to join me on this unconventional adventure. You are sure to find some promising revelations, challenges, and perhaps a healthier life on the other side.

As I document my experiences and share the research I have uncovered, "What if the path to optimal health is paved with… bacon?" I pose this question to you – the readers. I know it will challenge everything you thought you knew about food but buckle up.

Chapter 1: Are You Accidentally Poisoning Yourself with "Healthy" Food?

"What if that kale smoothie you're sipping is doing more harm than good?" This isn't just a question; I want you to reflect on it for a bit. What are the health benefits of Kale? What are the benefits of any "healthy" food? Before you shut down the arguments I am about to present, I want you to keep an open mind and dig deeper into the assumptions that have been spoon-fed to you by the media, the wellness industry, and even science itself.

Before we move ahead, let's take a step back and understand why certain plant foods came to be hailed as "superfoods." It wasn't always about their inherent nutritional value; instead, it was often the result of clever marketing strategies and selective scientific studies. The term "superfood" is widely used in discussions about food and health, but it lacks a specific definition in the scientific realm. While many superfoods claim positive health effects in studies, these findings may not always translate to real-world dietary benefits. In fact, a systematic review on the use of "superfoods" in marketing noted that there is no official regulation or scientific backing for the term, and the research behind many of these foods is often overstated.

In the early days, some foods were elevated to superfood status based on limited research and studies that were sometimes funded by the industries that benefited from their findings. For instance, kale was once just another leafy green and became a health icon almost overnight. Its rise to fame was fueled by its nutrient profile and savvy marketing campaigns that capitalized on the growing wellness trend. However, while kale contains important vitamins and minerals, it also contains high levels of oxalates, which can contribute to kidney stones in susceptible individuals.

The media played a significant role in shaping public perception. It often simplifies complex nutritional science into catchy headlines and buzzwords. These headlines, in turn, influenced consumer behavior and led to a widespread belief that consuming these "superfoods" was a direct path to better health. If you do a simple internet search for the word superfood, you will find close to 10 million results. All of these will be from predominantly health and health magazines, nutrition blogs, online newspapers, and nutritional supplement providers.

Often, the research these posts cite is preliminary and focused on specific populations, with findings that are not necessarily applicable to the general public. Despite this, the foods were marketed as universally beneficial to all people. This led to a skewed perception of what constitutes a healthy diet and what should be an essential part of our routine.

The Hidden World of Anti-nutrients

Let's introduce another buzzword for you to think about: **anti-nutrients**. These anti-nutrients are compounds found in plants that can interfere with the absorption of essential nutrients or cause digestive discomfort. They act as "roadblocks" in the body and hinder the absorption and utilization of vitamins and minerals. These compounds can be found in various plant-based foods and may affect how our body processes and absorbs nutrients from our diet.

Let's explore some of the most common anti-nutrients found in popular "health" foods:

Lectins: Lectins are proteins that bind to carbohydrates and can be found in high amounts in beans and grains. These naturally occurring compounds can disrupt digestion and interfere with nutrient absorption. It can potentially lead to gastrointestinal distress for some individuals.

Oxalates: Oxalates are organic compounds found in foods like spinach, kale, and nuts that can bind to calcium and other minerals in the digestive tract. It eventually forms crystals that may contribute to kidney stones. Think of these oxalates as "sponges" that soak up valuable minerals before your body can use them.

Phytates: Phytates, also known as phytic acid, are found in whole grains and legumes. These compounds can bind to minerals such as iron, zinc, and magnesium, reducing their bioavailability. These phytates are something like "locks" that keep essential nutrients trapped inside the food, making them harder for your body to unlock and use.

Goitrogens: Goitrogens are found in cruciferous vegetables like kale, broccoli, and Brussels sprouts and can interfere with thyroid function by disrupting iodine uptake. These Goitrogens would act like a "traffic jam" in the thyroid gland, where goitrogens slow down the normal processes that regulate metabolism. They can interfere with the thyroid, potentially leading to hypothyroidism in susceptible individuals.

Real-Life Stories of Dietary Change

There are many stories that various people have shared that emphasize the individuality of dietary needs. This means that what might work for you might not work for someone else. A user online shared his personal 21-day journey with a carnivore diet. He mentioned:

I'm not saying the carnivore diet is going to cure everything – there is no one-size-fits-all diet for everyone.

I just wanted to share my positive experience with the diet in hopes that I may inspire others who are already eating clean to jump into the carnivore diet.

Another example is Jake, a former natural bodybuilder who transitioned from a vegan diet to an animal-product-based diet during the 2020 lockdown. Despite initial reservations, he experienced remarkable improvements in his athletic performance and overall health. On his new diet of red meat, eggs, and salt, Jake found that he needed far fewer supplements and external sources of nutrition compared to his days as a vegan bodybuilder. His endurance levels soared, and he even completed a marathon after just three weeks of preparation.

Similarly, athletes like Adam Peaty, the men's 100m breaststroke world record holder, faced challenges when attempting a vegan diet. Peaty eventually returned to eating animal-based proteins to meet his demanding training needs as he struggled to maintain muscle mass on a vegan diet.

Brazilian sprinter Bruno Fratus also found that cutting out red meat and other animal-based foods hindered his performance, leading him to reintroduce them with great success at the Tokyo 2020 Olympics.

"I stopped cutting things. I stopped cutting red meat, fat, and white carbs like pasta," Fratus mentioned ahead of the Tokyo 2020.

"That's when I started to actually get stronger. My training quality increased drastically, I put good weight on in the weight room, and the quality of my sleep improved a lot," he continued while talking to Olympics.com.

This further reiterates the notion that there is no one perfect diet. We all need to evaluate our health and see which diet works best for us. One person online shared that they struggled with persistent digestive issues despite eating a diet rich in beans and whole grains. They only found relief after reducing their intake of foods high in lectins and phytates. Another person experienced worsening thyroid symptoms while consuming large amounts of kale and other cruciferous vegetables. Improvement was only seen after moderating their intake of these goitrogen-rich foods.

While anti-nutrients are a natural part of many plant foods, awareness and balance are key. I encourage you all reading this to listen to your bodies and consider that some of your "healthy" choices might need to be adjusted to better suit your needs.

Introducing the "Plant-based Troublemaker Detector"

Now that we better understand anti-nutrients, let me introduce you to another innovative and interactive tool, The Plant-based Troublemaker Detector. This tool is designed to help people identify potential problem foods in their diets that might contribute to unexplained symptoms or health issues. Allow me to walk you through a series of questions.

1. What symptoms are you experiencing?

2. How long have you been experiencing these symptoms?

3. Which of these foods do you consume regularly?

   - Soy products (tofu, tempeh, soy milk, etc.),

   - Gluten-containing grains (wheat, barley, rye, etc.)

   - Nuts and seeds

   - Nightshades (tomatoes, potatoes, peppers, etc.)

   - Legumes (beans, lentils, chickpeas, etc.)

   - Processed plant-based foods (mock meats, snacks, etc.)

   - Others

4. Have you recently introduced any new foods into your diet?

5. How would you describe your current stress levels?

By answering these questions, you will gain insights into which foods might be causing issues and how you can adjust your diet to feel your best.

This tool will act as a personalized guide and help you pinpoint specific foods that could be triggering adverse reactions, whether it's digestive distress, skin issues, or chronic fatigue.

Remember that an animal-product-based diet has been incredibly helpful to many people, especially athletes.

The Elimination Diet: A Personalized Approach

Once you identify the problem foods for yourself, you can take steps to eliminate or reduce them from your diet. The plant-based troublemaker detector can help you with the first part. Once you've identified potential culprits, you can monitor how your body responds when you stop eating those foods.

To help you out with the next step, let me introduce the Elimination Diet. The elimination diet involves removing potential trigger foods from the diet for a period of time. Then, you systematically reintroduce them to observe any adverse reactions. This method can be a powerful tool for identifying foods that may be causing health issues and are not best suited for you.

If you want to conduct your own elimination experiment, follow these steps:

1. Start by keeping a detailed food journal and note everything you eat and any symptoms you have experienced. This will help establish a baseline before you make any changes.

2. Then, start by removing common trigger foods—such as gluten, dairy, soy, nuts, and nightshades—from your diet for at least 2-4 weeks. During this period, your focus should be on eating simple, such as whole foods that are less likely to cause reactions.

3. After the elimination period, reintroduce one food at a time and observe how your body reacts over several days. This process helps to identify specific foods that may be causing issues for you. It also allows you to tailor your diet to your individual needs.

4. Finally, reflect on the results of their elimination diet and consider the physical and emotional impacts of the dietary changes. It is important to note that mental changes are just as important, if not more, than physical ones. This self-awareness will help you make informed decisions about which foods to include and avoid long-term.

Now that you have a better understanding and are equipped with practical tools and insights to take control of your health, you can uncover the hidden dietary culprits and make informed choices that align with your unique body and lifestyle.

There are various potential advantages of reducing or even eliminating plant foods for certain individuals. This is especially true for individuals grappling with autoimmune disorders, chronic inflammation, or persistent digestive issues. There is no truth in the statement that plant foods are always beneficial; for some, these foods might actually contribute to health problems.

While fruits, vegetables, and grains are often hailed as the foundation of a healthy diet, certain compounds found in these foods can be problematic. For example, in individuals with autoimmune conditions, these can sometimes act as triggers and set off immune responses that exacerbate symptoms.

Note that some people with autoimmune disorders have reported significant improvements in their condition after reducing or eliminating plant-based foods that contain these compounds.

Similarly, High-fiber foods—often recommended for digestive health- can be difficult to process for individuals with sensitive digestive systems and cause challenges for those with chronic digestive issues.

This happens because some plants' anti-nutrients and complex carbohydrates may cause discomfort, bloating, or other gastrointestinal symptoms. For these individuals, reducing the intake of plant foods that are high in fiber might offer relief and improve overall well-being.

But I must stress this approach is not a universal remedy. It may not be necessary for everyone. However, for those who have exhausted other dietary options without finding relief, the idea of cutting back on or eliminating certain plant foods could be worth exploring. Approach this concept as an experiment and listen to your body to determine what works best for YOU. Experimenting with your diet is a personal journey, and there's no harm in trying something new, especially if it could lead to better health and well-being. Before you dismiss the idea of reducing plants in your diet as crazy, ask yourself: What do you have to lose by experimenting? Your kale smoothie will still be there if you decide this isn't for you. But what if, like Jake, you discover a level of health you never thought possible?

Chapter 2: The Caveman's Revenge: Why Your Ancestors are Face-palming at Your Cornflakes Bowl

Imagine your Paleolithic ancestor watching you meticulously measure out a portion of Cornflakes. They'd probably grunt in confusion and offer you a mammoth steak instead. Your bowl of Cornflakes is the result of highly processed corn. Although corn has a good amount of nutrients, the processing grit strips off most of its nutrients. The milled corn is enhanced by adding back those essential nutrients, vitamins, minerals, malt, and sugar. Some brands even add artificial flavors, corn syrup, sugar, and honey. This only does more harm than good.

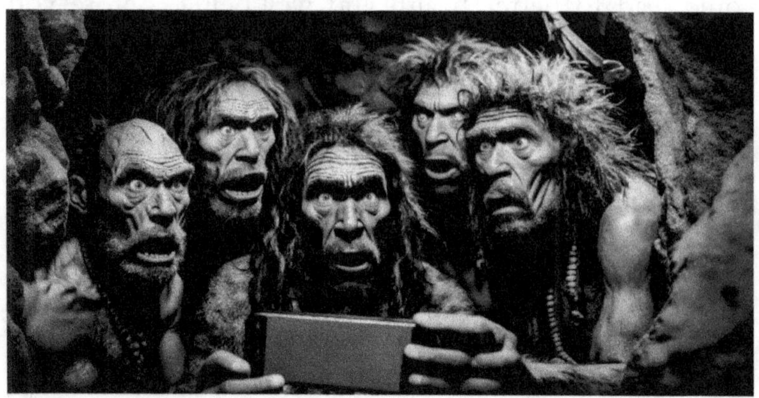

Although it's not something we learn often in school, the evolution of the human diet is a fascinating journey that spans millions of years.

The Evolutionary Timeline of the Human Diet

Our ancestors consistently consumed meat and used fire to cook as early as 2.6 million years ago. Initially, their diet was plant-based with some scavenging, but incorporating meat marked a significant evolutionary shift. During the Paleolithic era (2.6 million years ago to 10,000 BCE), humans were hunter-gatherers, relying on animal protein, fruits, and some plant-based foods, depending on seasonal availability. This radically changed with the Agricultural Revolution around 10,000 BCE, when humans transitioned to farming, which introduced grains, dairy, and other novel food sources.

Modern diets are a far cry from this ancestral fare. Industrialization and globalization have not only made processed foods more accessible but also distanced us from the nutrient-rich, unprocessed foods that supported human evolution for millions of years. Studies suggest that adopting a more "Stone Age" diet could significantly improve health outcomes by providing the nutrients our bodies evolved to process efficiently.

The early human groups hunted as a team and shared the rewards among the tribe. This communal approach to hunting increased the chances of a successful hunt and fostered strong social bonds and cooperation in our ancestors' harsh environments.

Carnivorous Traits in Human Anatomy

Recently, humans have been considered omnivores capable of consuming both plant and animal matter. However, several anatomical and physiological features of the human body suggest that we should have a diet that contains an increased amount of animal protein.

1. Digestive System Structure

For starters, the human digestive system provides evidence supporting the idea of humans having carnivorous traits. Our digestive tract has several features that align more closely with carnivorous mammals than with herbivores. For example, humans have a relatively shorter large intestine compared to obligate herbivores like cows or gorillas. This adaptation allows for efficient absorption of nutrients, particularly proteins and fats, which are more readily absorbed in the small intestine.

Similarly, herbivores' cecum is large and houses bacteria that help digest plant cellulose. Humans' cecum is much smaller. This reduction in cecum size suggests that our digestive system is not well-equipped for processing large quantities of plant fiber.

2. Tooth Morphology

Several features of Human teeth indicate adaptations for meat consumption. While our Canines are not as pronounced as lions or wolves, they are sharper and more pronounced than herbivores. These canines are useful for tearing food, particularly meat.

Similarly, human incisors are relatively flat and aligned in a way that is effective for biting into meat. Our premolars and molars are adapted to perform a simple function: shearing and crushing meat. Unlike herbivores' flat molars designed primarily for grinding plant material, our molars have a slightly raised cusp pattern suitable for an omnivorous diet that can handle plant fibers and meat.

The overall dental arcade shape in humans is more U-shaped than the more rounded or elongated shapes found in herbivores. This U-shape is efficient for processing varied foods, including tough meat fibers.

3. Stomach Acidity

Stomach acidity in humans is another physiological trait that hints at a carnivorous adaptation. The pH level of the human stomach is highly acidic and ranges from 1.5 to 3.5. This is similar to the stomach acidity found in primary carnivores, such as big cats. This highly acidic environment serves several purposes:

- **Protein Breakdown**: High acidity denatures proteins and makes it easier for enzymes like pepsin to break down into amino acids.

- **Pathogen Defense**: This acidity also acts as a barrier to pathogens commonly found in meat, including bacteria and parasites. This feature suggests that early humans might have consumed raw or minimally cooked meat, which required a robust acidic barrier to prevent infections.

The stomach's high acidity could also be an adaptation to a scavenging lifestyle. This suggests that the early humans might have consumed meat that was not always fresh and required a strong, acidic environment to neutralize potential pathogens.

4. Lack of Certain Digestive Enzymes for Plant Matter

Humans lack several enzymes necessary to digest certain types of plant material, such as:

- **Cellulase**: Humans do not produce cellulase, which is required to break down cellulose, a major component of plant cell walls. In contrast, many herbivores and some omnivores have either the enzyme cellulase or gut bacteria that produce it, allowing them to break down cellulose and extract energy from fibrous plants.

- **Phytases:** Humans also have a limited ability to digest phytates that are found in seeds, nuts, and grains, which can bind minerals and reduce their absorption. Phytate digestion requires Phytases, which are not present in significant amounts naturally in the human digestive system. This limitation further indicates that humans are not well-adapted to extract all possible nutrients from plant-based foods.

The Expensive Tissue Hypothesis

The **Expensive Tissue Hypothesis** [ETH] provides another clue to our carnivorous roots. Well, ETH is a concept related to brain and gut size in evolutionary biology. It suggests that for an evolved organism, there will be a tradeoff to accommodate a large brain without significantly increasing basal metabolic rate. Humans must use less energy on other expensive tissues like guts to have a larger brain. Our ancestors shifted to a meat-based diet that allowed them to develop larger brains without an unsustainable increase in overall metabolic rate. Since meat is a high-quality source of calories, fat, and protein, it provides concentrated energy that is easier and quicker to digest than fibrous plant material. It also provides more calories per unit weight, essential fatty acids, and amino acids that are vital for brain growth and function. This nutrient density means that less food needs to be consumed overall to meet nutritional needs. This reduces the burden on the digestive system.

This dietary change would have supported the energy demands of a growing brain without requiring a larger, more energy-consuming gut. This shift provided the necessary energy and nutrients to support the brain's growth and complexity. Had we not, we would have lacked the cognitive capabilities that now define modern humans.

Chemical Defenses in Plants

Let's also look at this from a common-sense standpoint. Plants are fixed to the ground by their roots and, therefore, can't escape predators. Many insects and animals will approach plants for a quick snack by munching on the leaves or stems. Plant leaves contain rich amounts of nutrients, carbohydrates, nitrogen, phosphorus, protein, and water, which the predators need and desire. That is why they are there, attempting to eat the plant.

However, plants have developed physical defenses such as bark, thorns, or thick leaves. Many plants contain chemicals that either taste bad or can harm predators. This "Chemical Protection" involves the production of compounds that can kill microbes and fungi. It has the potential to poison the predator or cause hallucinations. These chemical reactions are most concerning for modern humans. Although mass production, genetically modified organisms, and modern transportation allow greater access to plants and vegetables all year long, this comes with insecticides, fertilizers, and preservatives, which may ALL be harmful to our bodies.

Consuming only plant-based products is an "innovative" approach. If we look at different cultures, most traditional cultures thrive on heavily meat-based diets. Two of the most notable examples are the **Inuit** of the Arctic regions and the **Maasai** of East Africa. These groups have adapted to their unique environments and developed dietary practices that are much different than the American diet we know.

Traditional Meat-based Diets: Inuit and Maasai

1. The Inuit

The Inuit people inhabit the Arctic regions of Greenland, Canada, and Alaska. Their traditional diet is almost exclusively composed of animal products, and they have thrived on this diet for centuries.

The Inuit diet predominantly comprises marine animals like seals, whales, walruses, and fish. They also hunt land animals like caribou and birds. A significant portion of their diet comes from fatty animal parts, which provide the necessary calories and nutrients to survive in cold environments.

To maximize nutrient intake, the Inuit often consume raw or fermented food. I know, shocking, right? But this practice preserves vitamins that would otherwise be destroyed by cooking. For example, raw fish and seal meat are high in vitamin C, which prevents scurvy.

They also consume a high-fat diet, with around 50-75% of their calories coming from fats. However, these facts are primarily omega-3 fatty acids from marine sources, which have anti-inflammatory properties and are beneficial for heart health.

The traditional diet is low in carbohydrates. So naturally, their bodies rely on ketones as a primary energy source. Despite consuming a high-fat diet, the Inuit historically showed low rates of cardiovascular diseases. This could mainly be due to their high intake of omega-3 fatty acids, which help lower blood triglycerides and reduce the risk of clotting.

2. The Maasai

The Maasai are a semi-nomadic ethnic group inhabiting parts of Kenya and Tanzania and have a predominantly animal-based diet. They rely heavily on cattle and mainly consume milk and meat from cattle. Milk is a daily staple and provides a significant portion of their calories. Meat is consumed less frequently, typically during celebrations or ceremonies. Traditionally, they consume very few plant-based foods. Some wild herbs and plants are used for medicinal purposes, but their diet is overwhelmingly animal-based as it provides a sustainable source of nutrition without depleting the environment.

Both the Inuit and Maasai demonstrate how human populations have adapted to extreme environments with diets that defy conventional nutritional wisdom. This also proves that just because we are used to a certain diet does not mean it is the best one.

These cultural and traditional diets reiterate the idea that what we eat is highly personal and depends on our needs. All our bodies and environments differ drastically, so why shouldn't our diets?

For a long time, many people believed that early humans were primarily gatherers. They assumed we lived off nuts, fruits, and roots while occasionally scavenging for meat. However, recent archaeological evidence revealed that early humans were more adept hunters than previously thought, and that animal protein played a significant role in our diet. Let me debunk some myths for you:

Debunking Common Myths About Ancestral Diets

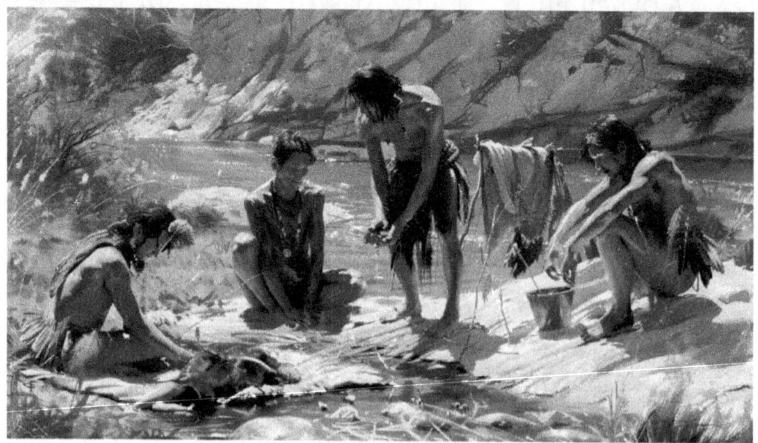

Myth #1: Our Ancestors Ate a "Paleo" Diet

The term "Paleo diet" often refers to a modern interpretation that includes lean meats, fish, fruits, vegetables, nuts, and seeds while excluding grains, legumes, and processed foods. However, early human diets varied significantly depending on geography, climate, season, and available resources. Since fruits and vegetables only grew during specific seasons and were not readily available at all times as they are now, most groups relied heavily on seafood. While others relied only on large or small game species. Meaning there was no single "Paleo" diet.

Myth #2: Our Ancestors Only Ate Raw Food

Cooking is an ancient practice. Evidence suggests that Homo erectus and perhaps even earlier hominins used fire to cook food as far back as 1.5 million years ago. Cooking makes food easier to digest, increases its caloric value, and reduces the risk of foodborne illnesses. It also breaks down plant toxins and makes certain nutrients more accessible. Archaeological findings do not support the assumption that our ancestors only consumed raw food.

Myth #3: Ancestral Diets Were Cholesterol-free

Many proponents of the "Paleo" diet assume that our ancestors consumed very little Cholesterol when, in reality, ancestral humans obtained about 35% of their dietary energy from fats, 35% from carbohydrates, and 30% from protein. Saturated fats contributed approximately 7.5% of total energy, and harmful trans-fatty acids were negligible. The Cholesterol consumption was substantial, perhaps around 480 mg per day. But again, the availability and consumption of carbohydrates would have varied greatly depending on the environment and season.

The Evolutionary Mismatch

Now that we've debunked some myths about ancestral diets, let's explore how our modern diet and lifestyle clash with our genetic programming. It is a fairly recent concept known as "Evolutionary Mismatch."

What is an Evolutionary Mismatch, you might ask? Well, an evolutionary mismatch occurs when the environment we live in changes faster than our bodies can adapt. This leads to a conflict between our genetic programming and our current lifestyle.

Modern humans face an **evolutionary mismatch**: our bodies are programmed for the lean, protein-rich diets of our ancestors, yet we now live in a world of processed, sugar-laden foods and sedentary lifestyles. This mismatch has contributed to the rise of lifestyle diseases like obesity, diabetes, and heart disease.

In terms of food and diets, our ancestors evolved in environments where food was scarce and physical activity was essential for survival. In contrast, modern society provides an abundance of high-calorie, processed foods and requires minimal physical exertion. This mismatch contributes to many health problems we see today, such as obesity, diabetes, and heart disease.

Unlike us, our ancestors ate a varied diet rich in lean proteins and healthy fats, with occasional high-energy foods. Today, we have access to processed foods high in sugars and refined grains, which were virtually nonexistent in the ancestral diet.

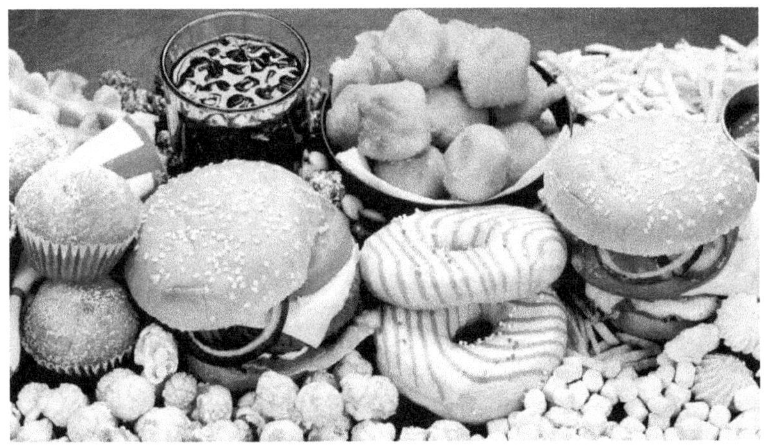

Our bodies are not well adapted to handle these new foods, leading to spikes in blood sugar and insulin resistance. Early humans had to be active daily to hunt, gather, and build shelter, which kept them fit and strong. Today, many of us sit for lengthy periods, leading to a host of health issues, including cardiovascular disease, musculoskeletal problems, and reduced metabolic health.

Before we discuss history further, let's play a fun game first. Simply answer these questions to see "How Well Do You Know Your Evolutionary Dietary History!"

1.What type of food was likely a primary source of calories for early humans living in the Arctic regions?

a) Berries and nuts

b) Fish and marine mammals

c) Tubers and roots

d) Grains and seeds

If you said fish and marine mammals, then you are correct. The Inuit relied heavily on marine life, which provided them with both calories and essential nutrients in a harsh climate where plant-based foods were scarce.

2. True or False: Early humans consumed only lean cuts of meat, avoiding fatty animal parts.

a) True

b) False

Answer: False. Early humans valued fatty parts of animals, such as bone marrow and organs, for their high caloric content and essential nutrients. It was crucial for survival in variable environments.

3. Which of the following is NOT a characteristic of the "Evolutionary Mismatch" concept?

a) Modern diets high in processed foods.

b) Sedentary lifestyles with minimal physical activity.

c) Genetically modified food enhancing nutrition.

d) Chronic stress from long-term exposure.

Genetically modified food-enhancing nutrition is the correct answer here. The concept of "Evolutionary Mismatch" focuses on how modern diets, sedentary lifestyles, and chronic stress differ from the conditions our ancestors evolved to thrive in, not on modern agricultural practices.

4. Which modern disease is most commonly associated with an evolutionary mismatch due to high sugar intake?

a) Scurvy

b) Diabetes

c) Tuberculosis

d) Arthritis

Say it with me, it's "Diabetes." High sugar intake, especially from processed foods, contributes to the development of insulin resistance and type 2 diabetes.

5. What did ancestral populations use as a common food preservation method?

a) Refrigeration

b) Fermentation

c) Microwaving

d) Freezing

Fermentation was a common method for preserving food, allowing it to last longer and making some nutrients more accessible, such as in fermented fish, meats, or dairy.

All of the information we have discussed so far points in one direction: if our ancestors thrived on a meat-based diet for millions of years, is it possible that our current nutritional guidelines have led us astray? Perhaps it's time to consider that the 'caveman diet' wasn't so primitive after all.

Chapter 3: The Protein Paradigm Shift: Building a Better You, One Steak at a Time

Forget everything you thought you knew about protein. It's time for a meaty revelation that might just change your life—and your biceps.

Think of your body as an extremely complicated machine, akin to a high-tech robot. Just as a robot needs many parts to run, like gears and wires, your body requires proteins to function. Proteins are the raw materials used to build and maintain every part of the body, from its structure to its critical functions.

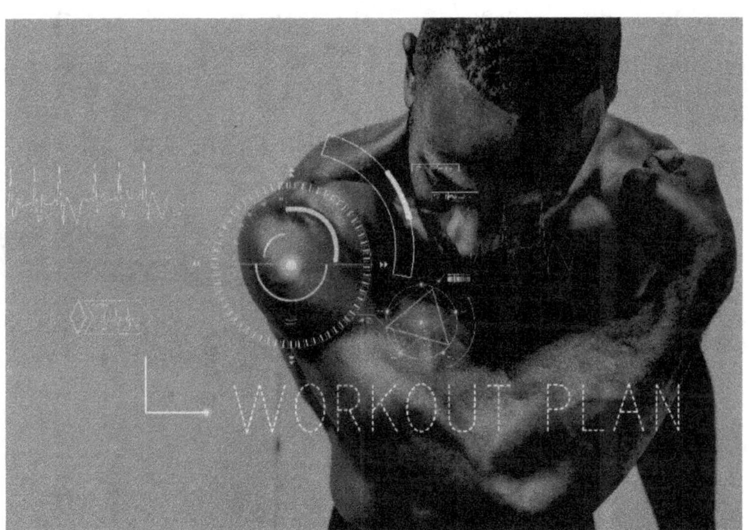

The Building Blocks of Life

Proteins are large, complex molecules composed of small units called amino acids. Amino acids could be thought of as the LEGO bricks of proteins; much like how LEGO bricks come in many shapes and colors for different structures, amino acids have unique properties depending upon what they do, such as building and repairing tissues, making hormones, and so on.

There are 20 amino acids classified as either essential or non-essential. The body can synthesize non-essential amino acids, but essential amino acids must be obtained from the diet. Of the nine essential amino acids—histidine, isoleucine, leucine, lysine, methionine, phenylalanine, threonine, tryptophan, and valine—animal-based foods provide a complete package of all the amino acids your body needs.

Essential amino acids must be taken through what we eat. This means that proteins are involved in almost every single process related to the functioning of human physiology.

Complete Vs. Incomplete Proteins

Now, let's take a closer look at complete versus incomplete proteins using an analogy of a set of LEGOs.

Think of complete proteins as a sort of LEGO set: it comes with all the pieces one needs to build a specific model. An important aspect of meat is that it contains all nine essential amino acids in the right proportions your body needs. Animal-based proteins, including those in meat, fish, eggs, and dairy products, are similar to these all-inclusive LEGO sets. They contain all the "pieces" required for your body to perform optimally.

Incomplete proteins (non-essential), on the other hand, are missing pieces from LEGO sets. Most proteins in plants, including beans, lentils, nuts, and whole grains, do not contain one or more of the essential amino acids in their proper proportions. This means one would need to combine two types of plant-based foods to cover all the essential amino acids. An example would be beans combined with rice or nuts with whole grains to provide a full protein profile. Quinoa and soy are exceptions in this case, as they contain all nine essential amino acids. Soy contains phytoestrogens, particularly isoflavones, which are plant compounds that can mimic estrogen in the body. They do not contain actual estrogen hormones but can have estrogen-like effects due to their ability to bind to estrogen receptors.

An important constituent of any diet, protein provides many uses, helping keep your body's complex machinery running smoothly. In a carnivore diet, you can usually get all the essential amino acids, but vegetarians and vegans have difficulty consuming protein because different plant-based protein sources contain different essential amino acids. Putting it all together, proteins are the LEGO building blocks of your body: they build, maintain, and repair its structure and functions. Knowing the differences in types of proteins, whether complete or incomplete, allows one to make better choices for maintaining all body machinery.

Protein Quality: The Key to Optimal Health

When we think of protein, we often think of muscle building, but protein does so much more for the body. It repairs tissues, produces enzymes and hormones, supports the immune system, and powers brain function. In terms of quality, protein is judged by its biological value (BV), protein efficiency ratio (PER), and net protein utilization (NPU). These metrics measure how well the body uses the protein for growth, repair, and overall functioning.

For example, animal proteins tend to have higher BV, PER, and NPU than plant proteins, meaning they're more efficiently utilized by the body. This is why protein from meat and animal sources can provide your body with optimal performance, just like the best parts fuel a high-performance sports car.

Biological Value (BV) is a measure of how effectively your body utilizes a protein source. Now, think of the car's efficiency in using fuel and converting it into performance. A protein with high BV provides much of the essential amino acids in appropriate ratios that your body can easily use. Generally speaking, animal-based proteins are likely to have a high BV because they usually contain abundant essential amino acids.

The Protein Efficiency Ratio [PER] is just like checking the fuel efficiency of your car. It is a measure of how a protein is efficiently utilized by the body to produce growth, according to intake. For instance, if two kinds of proteins are being consumed, PER will help determine which is more potent in growth and development. Proteins with high PERs help build and maintain your muscles more.

Net Protein Utilization [NPU] is the analysis of how well the overall system of the car runs using that fuel to perform; more accurately, it is the percentage of utilized ingested protein by your body for growth and repair. An NPU is higher when more of the consumed protein is utilized instead of wasted.

Now, let's talk about essential amino acids. Think of yourself building some sort of high-tech gadget and think there are crucial components you'd have to possess for it to function. Well, the essential amino acids are just those crucial components because you cannot make a gadget without them. It is called "essential" because your body cannot produce the amino acid on its own, and it must be obtained through your diet.

Why are they important? The amino acids in your diet provide the raw material your body needs to build and repair tissues, synthesize enzymes and hormones, and carry out many other critical functions. Just as the building blocks of a house are, if some of those essential amino acids aren't available to your body, that puzzle of higher function will never fully come into being.

My Personal Transformation

I remember a time when I felt sluggish and unfocused. After consulting with a nutritionist, I increased my intake of complete proteins like eggs, fish, and steak. Within weeks, my energy surged, and my mind became clearer. My body relaxed as inflammation was reduced and anxieties subsided. My "engine" had been fueled with the right protein, and the results were transformative. This ultimately led to a reduction in my high blood pressure.

This isn't just my experience. I came across a testimonial from someone following the carnivore diet, a 50-year-old male who was battling type 2 diabetes, arthritis, and chronic fatigue. After starting the carnivore diet, his blood sugar stabilized, his inflammation disappeared, and his energy returned. He lost over 60 pounds in just 90 days. The only change? He switched to a diet focused on high-quality animal protein.

"I am a 50-year-old male with a starting weight of 303.13 lbs. I have type 2 diabetes with blood sugar at 176.4 mg/dL, as well as arthritis, fibromyalgia, chronic fatigue syndrome, brain fog, post-exertion malaise, adult-onset asthma, sleep apnea, and inflammation issues. Due to my weight, my heart and lungs were compressed when I lay down.

"I started the Carnivore diet on August 6th, 2023. By day 4, my blood sugar dropped to 95.4 mg/dL, and my inflammation was gone. By day 7, the arthritis and fibromyalgia pain had disappeared. By day 14, my brain fog was gone, my energy levels were up, chronic fatigue was less, sleep apnea had disappeared, and asthma symptoms were reduced.

"Throughout this, I was losing weight rapidly, about 5 lbs. per week. On day 100, I had full blood work done. My testosterone was high, vitamin D and iron levels were normal, and all levels were in the healthy range. I weighed 242.51 lbs. and had lost 60.63 lbs. in 90 days.

"My doctor then revealed that my body was producing and managing insulin levels completely on its own again, and I was no longer diabetic. My doctor was amazed and relieved for me. All of this positive change was because I only ate a large beef or lamb steak for each evening meal, with Redmond's Real Salt

and a 1cm thick cut of grass-fed butter on top of the steak, cooked in a non-stick, non-toxic pan.

"Sometimes, I ate eggs. I had cut out all fruit, vegetables, carbs, sugars, sweeteners, processed foods, legumes, sauces, spices, pepper, cooking oils, seed oils, milk, soft drinks, juices, and tea. I still drank coffee (brew and instant) with added butter and salt. I would wholeheartedly recommend the Carnivore diet to any person suffering from chronic health conditions or diabetes."

This example suggests that all the misconceptions about the carnivore diet are baseless. Speaking of baseless Myths, let's dispel some common protein myths.

Dispelling Protein Myths

Myth 1: High-protein Diets are Inherently Dangerous

This may well be the most pervasive myth. While it is true that a very excessive intake of protein, especially from sources with heavy processing, has its negative repercussions, normally balanced diets that contain just the right amount of protein intake would not pose any problem for the majority. High-protein diets can support muscle growth and weight management when correctly applied.

Myth 2: You Must Eat Protein at Every Meal

Some people think they have to have some protein at each meal for health's sake. Protein is not a problem nutrient, and your body is quite adept at using protein throughout the day. As long as you get a balanced protein intake through your meals, you'll be fine.

Just keep in mind that most plant-based proteins are incomplete, and a combination of various plant sources is required to achieve the amount of all amino acids necessary for your body. Not to mention that plant-based proteins often lack other beneficial stuff.

In other words, knowledge about protein quality helps you make good choices about what to eat so your body will have the best fuel possible. Do not let myths lead you away from making a superior food choice. Whether you order prime ribeye steak or seafood broil for lunch, protein is part of every meal and can pump up an appetite.

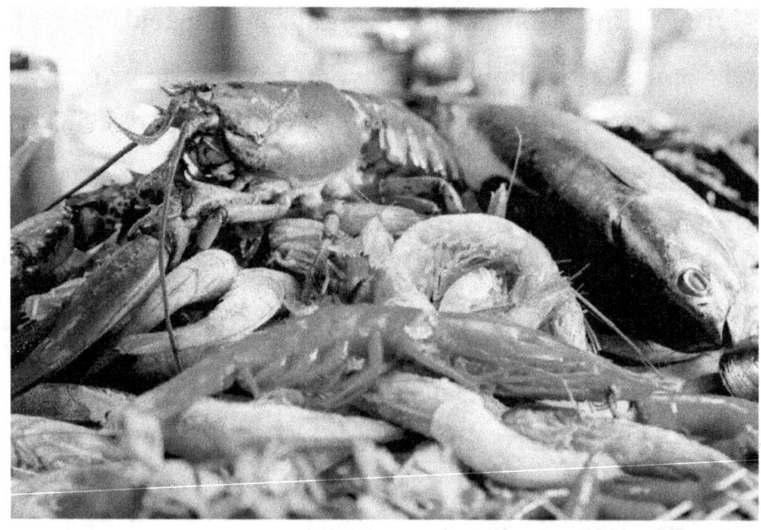

Now, think of lunch prior to starting an animal-based diet. Perhaps you started with a nice salad and a glass of sweet tea. You finish the salad but are still feeling hungry. You have some bread, but that does not quite satisfy your hunger, either. A nice sandwich with more bread, cheese, vegetables, condiments, and deli meat will surely fulfill your appetite. You may not realize that your body's quest for protein has just caused you to overindulge in non-animal-based foods, which could lead to weight gain.

The Protein Leverage Hypothesis

One fascinating concept to consider is the Protein Leverage Hypothesis, which suggests that our bodies have a genetic target for protein intake, and if this is not met, it may over-consume the other macronutrients, carbohydrates, and fats to satisfy that urge. The Protein Leverage Hypothesis suggests that the human body has a specific protein target that it seeks to meet.

When we don't consume enough protein, the theory proposes that our bodies may drive us to eat more carbohydrates and fats in an attempt to satisfy this target. That's the reason many end up overconsuming calories and why high-protein diets appear to cause a drop in total calorie intake and improved weight management.

This hypothesis is interesting in the context of the obesity epidemic.

If diets are low in protein, we may overeat on a total basis; high-protein diets allow us to reach our protein targets in fewer calories, give us better weight control, and reduce desires to snack on excess carbohydrates and fats.

The Many Functions of Protein

While many people associate protein with building muscles, the protein has a lot more functions in the body. Here is a closer look at the many different ways protein takes part in the body:

1. Immune System Function

Proteins help to build a healthy immune system. Antibodies are one of the special types of proteins that assist in identifying and neutralizing any bacteria, viruses, or other germs that may invade your body. If your protein intake is deficient, ultimately, it weakens your immunity system and makes you prone to diseases.

2. Production of Hormones

It is also an integral part of hormone production. Hormones, such as insulin and thyroid hormones, basically involve proteins in the regulation of most bodily functions, ranging from the sugar level in your blood to metabolism. This is the reason a deficiency of protein knocks these hormonal balances off-kilter and, on the whole, reduces health and well-being.

3. Production of Enzymes

Enzymes are types of proteins that act as catalysts for biochemical reactions in the body. From digestion in the gut to helping various cellular processes, enzymes play an important role in keeping all activities running smoothly. If protein intake is insufficient to sustain this, enzyme production is impaired, adversely affecting digestion and many other vital functions.

4. Tissue Repair

This helps the tissues maintain and repair themselves. Protein builds up again whenever one gets a cut or even strained muscles. For this reason, proteins are essential for athletes and anyone recovering from injuries or surgeries.

5. Brain Function

Protein also plays a vital role in the functioning of the brain. Neurotransmitters, the chemicals that essentially transmit signals in the brain, often stem from amino acids made by proteins. Sufficient intake of protein aids in good cognitive function, mood regulation, and mental clarity in general.

Now that we understand the importance of proteins, it's time for you to incorporate them into your diet. I am presenting a week-long protein quality tracking challenge in steps; this will help you better understand your protein intake and start researching the benefits of higher-quality proteins:

A Week-long Protein Quality Challenge

Day 1: Assess Your Current Protein Intake

1. 1.Start by keeping a detailed food diary for the day and writing down everything you eat and drink. Be sure to pay special attention to recording sources of protein.

2. Establish whether your source of protein, such as animal proteins, is complete or incomplete, which includes mostly those from plants.

Day 2: Assessing Protein Quality

1. Using tools or application software based on a protein quality index will help in ascertaining the quality of your source of proteins. Look for values and measures such as Biological Value, Protein Efficiency Ratio, and Net Protein Utilization. There are various apps available on the market to track your protein intake, some of which are Protein Pal: Protein Tracker and Hello Protein-Protein Tracker.

2. Observe if your diet lacks complete proteins or identifies any gaps in essential amino acids.

Day 3: Set Protein Goals

1. Based on your activity level, muscle-building goals, and weight management, among others, determine your daily protein needs.

2. Develop meals with the inclusion of high-quality proteins. High-quality proteins include lean meats, dairy, eggs, and/or other food sources that include all essential amino acids.

Day 4: Complete Proteins

1. Consume at least one source of complete protein in every meal.

2. Observe how this adjustment impacts your level of hunger, energy, and how you feel in general.

Day 5: Check-in and Adjust

1. Reflect on how you feel to gauge if your energy is different, whether you have mental or if you feel like you are performing at a good physical level.

2. Continue with your protein intake for today, making any additional adjustments according to your feelings and needs.

Day 6: Get Feedback

1. If possible, have a nutritionist or a dietician review your protein intake and the quality of it. They will be able to make more personalized recommendations and adjustments.

Day 7: Review and Reflect

1. Go back and look at your food diary and your notes from this past week. Reflect on how increasing the quality of your protein intake has affected overall health and satisfaction.

2. Determine how you will continue to include high-quality proteins in your diet from now on.

In short, knowledge of the Protein Leverage Hypothesis and protein's multifaceted roles in the body empower individuals with informed dietary choices. One can upgrade this diet to the next level for improved health and well-being by paying attention to and experimenting with protein quality and variety. It's time to shift your protein paradigm. Your ancestors built civilization on the power of animal protein. Shifting your focus toward high-quality animal protein can be transformative for your health. By learning about protein's many roles, from supporting your immune system to enhancing brain function, you'll discover how to build a stronger, healthier you—one steak at a time.

Chapter 4: The Fat Redemption: From Dietary Villain to Metabolic Hero

Ladies and gentlemen of the dietary jury, before you stand the defendant, who has long been the subject of criticism—fat. This nutrient has been wrongly accused and unjustly vilified for decades, but now it's time to vindicate fat!

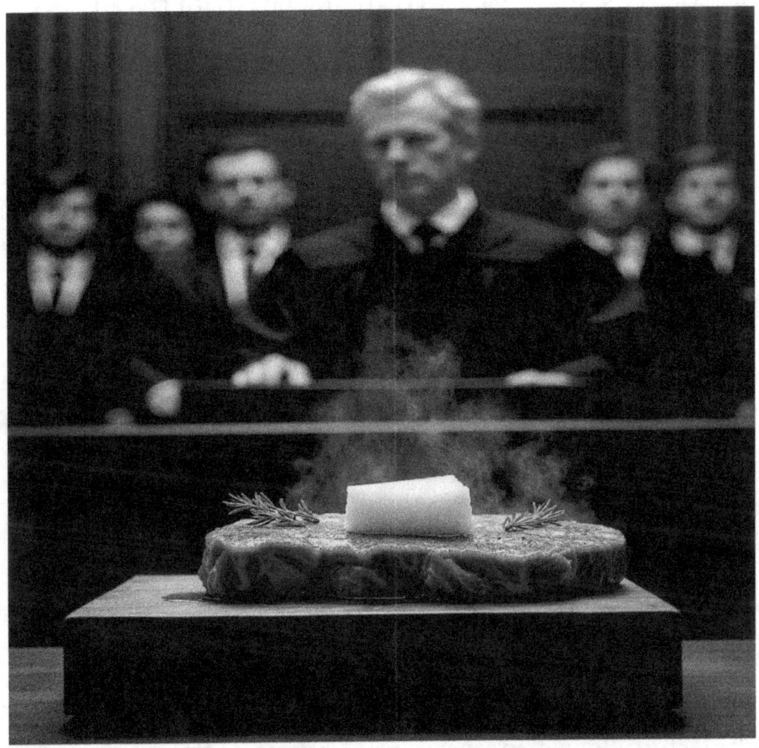

Let me take you to the commencement of this warped tale, a real detective story, if there was one. Picture it: the early 1950s, a smoke-filled room where science and politics mixed like bourbon and soda. This is where our story starts, with a man named Ancel Keys and his infamous Seven Countries Study.

Keys was no ordinary gumshoe. He was a scientist with a hunch, a man who believed that fat, that silky smooth substance, was the chief villain behind heart disease. His study followed the dietary patterns in seven countries and apparently showed the more saturated fat one consumed, the higher the prevalence of heart disease. Well, the town was abuzz. Headlines trumpeted, "Fat is the Enemy!" And with that, the low-fat frenzy got underway and ushered in many nutritional myths to follow that would create dietary choices for decades.

Keys backed his hypothesis with his research and observations that populations in regions like southern Italy and Greece, where people followed what is now called the Mediterranean diet (rich in fruits, vegetables, fish, and olive oil), had much lower rates of heart disease. He popularized this diet as a healthy lifestyle choice. Keys strongly advocated for the idea that high levels of dietary saturated fats and cholesterol contribute to elevated blood cholesterol levels, increasing the risk of heart disease. This hypothesis influenced public health policies on fat consumption. Critics later pointed out flaws in Keys' research, like cherry-picking the data, which led to over-simplifying the relationship between saturated fat and heart disease.

But let us not get ahead of ourselves. We wouldn't have a complete story without meeting the suspects, and each type of fat has something different to say.

We should start with the main character of the story, **Saturated Fat** (The Big Villain). Think of this fat as a burly, no-nonsense detective who would always have a cigar hanging from his lips. With his rough exterior and refusal to budge, this would be your classic bad guy. He's found in red meats, butter, and full-fat dairy products. Together with the Seven Countries Study, this earned him a poor reputation as a lead suspect in the crime of heart disease. With its rigid structure, Saturated Fat apparently contributes to the blockage of arteries. He is the strong-armed force behind it all.

Next up is **Monounsaturated Fat (The Smooth Talker)**. Conversely, Monounsaturated Fat is smooth, debonair, and a sly smooth talker. Just picture him in his well-fitted suit, sipping a glass of fine olive oil. He is the hero of this story and hides in avocados, nuts, and olive oil. Monounsaturated Fat smooths out the edges and helps reduce bad cholesterol, Romeo to your heart's well-being. He is the one who says, "Chill, I've got it," while he balances things out.

Now comes the extroverted and creative **Polyunsaturated Fat (The Innovator)**, one who is always wearing the latest gadgets in the medical world. The guy who loves smartphone accessories is all about that edge. Think omega-3 and omega-6 fatty acids found in fatty fish, flaxseeds, and walnuts; he's known to have this knack for reducing inflammation and supporting brain health. As the forward thinker he is, Polyunsaturated Fat keeps updating himself through constant change, making the body run like an oiled machine.

Up next, we have the **Trans Fat (Slippery Felon)**. It is the slippery two-faced character in this story. He's the one hiding in all those highly processed foods and baked goods and whose smile doesn't quite seem to reach his eyes. A little underhandedly, Trans Fat derives its structure through hydrogenation to stay solid at room temperature. He's linked to a spate of health woes, ranging from heart disease to inflammation, and is seemingly the ultimate villain that's been eluding everyone.

As the years rolled by, the low-fat craze began to take its toll. What had been a narrative born from scientific suspicion mushroomed out of control into full-blown diet dogma. Then, as new research emerged, it became clear that the story wasn't as simple as a one-dimensional villain. It was later uncovered that saturated fat wasn't singularly at fault, and trans-fat proved to be the real mastermind of mischief.

As we worked our way through the grand unraveling of this nutritional whodunit, we unraveled the fact that not all fats were considered equal. Each one was playing a role, and the plot thickened. The case was nowhere near closed, but the shadows did begin to clear.

The next time you sit down to a meal, remember that each of the characters in this tale has a role to play. And as the villainy of Trans Fat may be self-evident, Saturated, Monounsaturated, and Polyunsaturated Fats, all play their parts in the grand drama known as nutrition. Keep your wits about you; you will make your way through the dietary maze with more confidence.

There were many poor outcomes of the low-fat craze of the '70s and '80s, like margarine - "I can't believe it's not butter" which offered a *lite* version of butter but introduced soy oils high in omega-6 and skim milk, which removed beneficial animal fats.

We are about to discuss the affair against our old adversary, Fat, who is accused of numerous crimes against human health.

This case has riveted public attention for decades, with allegations running from heart disease to obesity. But today, we pull back the veil on this high-profile trial and take a closer look at the truth about Fat's role in our bodies. Let's start with the membrane.

Physiological Roles of Fat

1. **Cell Membrane Structure:** Consider the cell membrane as the ultimate fortress, protecting the secrets inside. Cell membranes made up of fat ensure cells communicate effectively with each other. Fat, in the form of phospholipids, would be considered the bricks within this wall. As such, the lipids form a double layer, hence a flexible and tough barrier that controls what enters and what does not enter the cell. Without this protective layer, our cells would easily be prone to destruction and malfunction.

2. **Synthesis of Steroid Hormones:** Think of Fat as a chemist in the lab, whipping up vital hormones. Steroid hormones, which include estrogen and testosterone, are manufactured from a form of fat known as cholesterol. **Cholesterol** is a type of fat, called lipid, which is converted into **pregnenolone** at the site of mitochondria within cells. Pregnenolone is then responsible for producing all steroid-based hormones. A balanced intake of fats is crucial for hormonal balance, especially for women, where too low fat can disrupt menstrual cycles.

Starting from pregnenolone follows a series of enzymatic reactions that eventually lead to the production of various hormones such as Testosterone, the primary male sex hormone, although present in females but only in smaller amounts, and Estrogen, the primary female sex hormone, which includes estradiol, estrone, and estriol.

These hormones, elaborated in large amounts, attend to some rudimentary physiological processes, such as reproductive health, stress response, and more. Fat is the invisible hand conducting a symphony of functions here.

3. Nutrient Absorption: Fat is an important carrier in the process of absorption of fat-soluble vitamins A, D, E, and K. Had it not been for fat, these much-needed nutrients in the body would just be washed away, slipped into our system without being let out just like a fugitive. To understand how fat helps absorb fat-soluble vitamins, take a look at the following evidence:

When you consume foods containing fat-soluble vitamins, they mix with dietary fat in the stomach and small intestine. The presence of fat triggers the release of bile from the liver and pancreatic enzymes. Bile helps emulsify fats, breaking them down into smaller droplets, which makes them more accessible for absorption.

Then, the fat-soluble vitamins (A, D, E, and K) are absorbed along with the fat droplets through the lining of the small intestine. Fat-soluble vitamins impact bone health (vitamin D) and blood clotting (vitamin K). Once inside the intestinal cells, these vitamins are incorporated into chylomicrons (fat transport molecules) and transported through the lymphatic system into the bloodstream. Keep in mind that unlike water-soluble vitamins, which are excreted if not used, fat-soluble vitamins are stored in the body's fatty tissues and liver. They can be released when the body needs them.

4. Brain Function: Like in the courtroom of the mind, Fat is the unsung hero. Highly content with fat, the brain requires fats, especially omega-3 fatty acids, to function optimally. These help maintain neuronal membrane integrity and support cognitive function, including memory, concentration, and reduced inflammation. Without such kinds of fats, the brain acts like a rusting machine unable to cope with everyday life. There is emerging research connecting omega-3s to reducing the risk of neurodegenerative diseases like Alzheimer's.

While they can be found in both plant and animal sources, several animal-based foods are particularly rich in these beneficial fats, especially in the form of EPA (eicosapentaenoic acid) and DHA (docosahexaenoic acid), which are the most bioavailable forms of omega-3s for the body.

The foods that are excellent sources of Omega-3 Fatty Acids are the following: salmon (especially wild-caught), mackerel, sardines, anchovies, herring, tuna (especially albacore tuna), shellfish, oysters, mussels, crab, and shrimp.

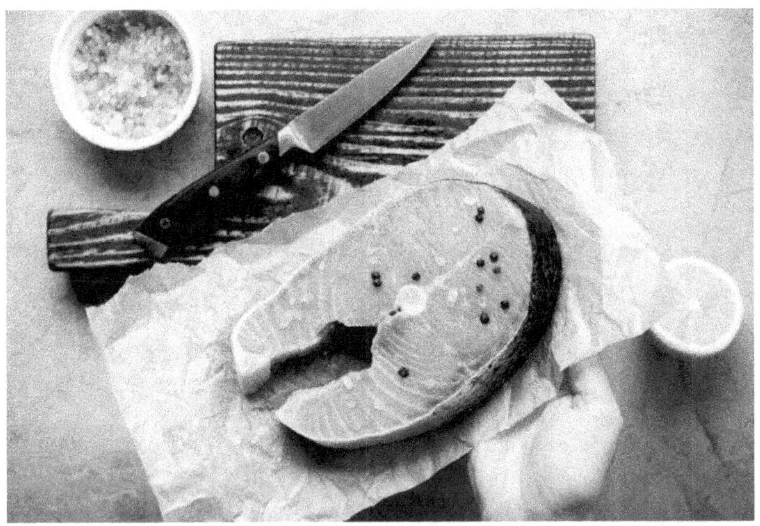

Cod Liver Oil is another such food—although not a direct food—it is a potent source of omega-3 fatty acids and contains vitamins A and D.

Grass-fed meat and dairy are not as high in omega-3s as fish; grass-fed beef contains higher levels of omega-3s compared to conventionally grain-fed beef. Milk, cheese, and butter from grass-fed cows have a better omega-3 to omega-6 ratio, with more omega-3 content. Omega-3-enriched eggs are another great source of protein. Chickens that are fed a diet rich in omega-3s, often including flaxseed, have higher levels of omega-3s than regular eggs.

Pasture-raised eggs also tend to have more omega-3s compared to conventionally raised eggs, though to a lesser extent than omega-3-enriched eggs.

Incorporating these animal foods into your diet is a good way to ensure you're getting adequate amounts of EPA and DHA, which are crucial for brain function, heart health, and reducing inflammation.

5. Energy Storage and Production: Fat acts as the repository of energy supply within the body. When glucose is in short supply, Fat mobilizes to produce energy. Hence, it undergoes a process known as lipolysis, whereby the fatty acids produced by it are released and can be burned for fuel. Similar to maintaining a savings bank account, Fat is very important for keeping reserves to fall back upon when times are lean. While on the Carnivore Diet, there is no intake of sugar or carbohydrates; thus, the fats become the energy for the body. This shift to fat-burning in ketosis can also help regulate insulin and blood sugar levels, which further promotes fat's role in metabolic health.

Well, for a long time, the prosecution has pointed a finger at Saturated Fat as the chief culprit in heart disease. Now, new evidence has come to light that could absolve our defendant. Lately, meta-analyses[1] have begun to challenge the data that incriminates saturated fat for

---

[1] Malhotra A, Redberg RF, Meier P. Saturated fat does not clog the arteries: coronary heart disease is a chronic inflammatory condition, the risk of which can be effectively reduced from healthy lifestyle interventions, *British Journal of Sports Medicine* 2017;51:1111-1112.

causing heart disease. Some have concluded that the association may be less straightforward than had been previously thought. Indeed, the evidence shows that other factors like refined carbohydrates and overall diet quality play significant roles.

Moreover, new studies[2] suggest genetic predisposition can affect the way people react to saturated fat. As it were, many people may metabolize saturated fat differently, defying the one-size-fits-all wisdom that has shaped dietary advice for decades. Diets high in fruits, vegetables, and whole grains reduce potential risks that are said to be linked with saturated fat. It's not just the fat in and of itself but the context of the whole diet.

In its defense, it will be said and believed that even if Saturated Fat isn't the ultimate villain, then the real culprit may well be the processed foods and refined sugars that come along with it. Ladies and gentlemen, it is now the turn of all of you to take to the stand. Step in and interact with your guide on:

Decoding Your Body's Fat-burning Signals

1. Does your energy remain consistent throughout the day? If your body uses fat for fuel, you might

---

[2] Vesnina A, Prosekov A, Kozlova O, Atuchin V. Genes and Eating Preferences, Their Roles in Personalized Nutrition. Genes (Basel). 2020 Mar 27;11(4):357. doi: 10.3390/genes11040357. PMID: 32230794; PMCID: PMC7230842.

have much more sustained energy without spiking and crashing from those sugar highs and lows.

2. Are you feeling sharper mentally or more focused? A diet that's supportive of fat metabolism will sharpen your cognitive function, especially when the fats are healthy, such as omega-3s.

3. Are your cravings for sweet treats fewer and farther between? When your body is efficiently burning fat for fuel, the number of cravings you have may lessen since fat serves as a longer-lasting energy source.

The judgment is far from being delivered, but one thing is for sure: Fat is not the straightforward bad guy it once had been made out to be. It plays a crucial role in our bodies, and a balanced understanding of its functions and effects can lead to better health outcomes.

As we close this courtroom drama, remember that the truth about fat is more subtle than the 'guilty' or 'not guilty' verdict. Bring to your diet the wisdom of recent research and the awareness of how your body interacts with different types of fat. The case for a balanced and informed nutrition approach has never been so clear.

Ladies and gentlemen, fasten your seat belts as we go on a fantastic ride of metabolism next. Consider your body as one high-octane motor that has just revved its engine on fuel that may give it turbocharged performance or one that would stall it altogether. Today, we talk about the ketogenic state-a radical fuel switch that reboots your body for ultimate performance.

Changing fuels is not a light matter in the world of automobiles. Imagine your car on gasoline, purring marvelously. Suddenly, imagine retrofitting it to run on diesel. It's a whole new ballgame, but it comes with distinct advantages. And it fits precisely into what we're discussing here.

On a standard high-carb diet, your body is powered mainly by glucose, or in our case, gasoline for all essential purposes. Glucose is a quick, readily available energy, but like all high-octane fuels, it spikes and dives into energy levels. When you go onto a ketogenic diet, you flip over to using fat as your energy source, which is a more stable, efficient type of energy—almost like putting diesel fuel in your car.

The Ketogenic State

When in a ketogenic state, a transformation occurs in your body. With no glucose available, your liver breaks down fat into small molecules called ketones. And now those ketones have just become new fuel for you, actually sustaining longer-term energy. Make this switch from fuel, and you will experience a number of potential advantages.

1. Unlike glucose, whose intake leads to energy highs followed by debilitating energy crashes, ketones keep energy levels in a tightly controlled area. This may result in increased stamina and endurance, particularly with prolonged physical activities.

2. Many people find their mental focus is sharper and have improved cognitive function when in ketosis. Ketones are the best, or likely a clean and efficient energy source for the brain. As noted through research, it allows for better mental clarity and fewer instances of brain fog.

3. The magical ketogenic diet can help with weight loss by increasing fat utilization and reducing hunger. Thus, through fat as an energy source, managing appetite can be easier to control.

4. Since your body is dependent on fat as a fuel source, you no longer require all that glucose, which leads to balanced blood sugar levels and increased insulin sensitivity.

5. Less inflammation accompanied by a reduction in blood sugar and insulin levels as the ketogenic diet drastically reduces carbohydrate intake, leading to lower blood glucose levels and, consequently, lower insulin levels.

High blood sugar and insulin spikes are common within diets that are high in refined carbs. Therefore, it can trigger inflammatory responses in the body. Reducing these glucose fluctuations helps decrease inflammation, which helps with metabolic conditions like insulin resistance and type 2 diabetes.

Ketones (produced during ketosis) are a cleaner fuel source for the body compared to glucose. They produce fewer reactive oxygen species (ROS), which are byproducts of metabolism that can cause oxidative stress and inflammation.

Inflammation and the Keto Diet

Studies show that a ketogenic diet can lower levels of inflammatory markers like C-reactive protein (CRP), TNF-alpha, and interleukin-6 (IL-6). These markers are associated with chronic inflammation and are linked to conditions like heart disease, arthritis, and autoimmune disorders.

AGEs are compounds that form when proteins or fats combine with sugars in the bloodstream. A diet high in sugar and refined carbs leads to the formation of more AGEs, which can contribute to inflammation and oxidative stress. By minimizing carbohydrate intake, a ketogenic diet reduces the formation of AGEs, helping to lower inflammation. Many people on a ketogenic diet emphasize whole, unprocessed foods, including healthy fats, leafy greens, and low-carb vegetables. These foods are rich in antioxidants, which help fight inflammation. Additionally, avoiding processed foods, refined sugars, and unhealthy fats (such as trans fats) reduces inflammation.

Here is the striking contrast in diet styles:

High-carb diets tend to spike blood sugar, leading to more frequent inflammation, whereas low-carb diets tend to stabilize blood sugar and reduce inflammation

Some research suggests that a carnivore diet can help balance gut bacteria by promoting a healthier microbiome. A diet high in refined carbs and sugars can cause imbalances in gut flora, leading to increased intestinal permeability (leaky gut), which can promote systemic inflammation. By reducing processed foods and carbs, the keto diet may support better gut health and reduce inflammation linked to gut issues.

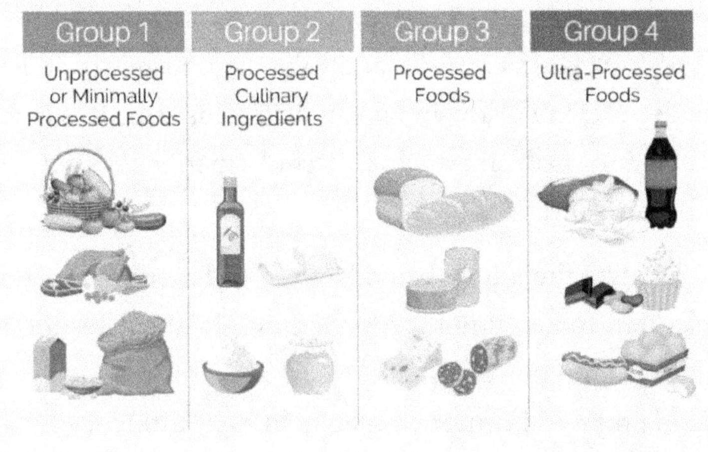

Carnivore diets are effective for weight loss, particularly in reducing visceral fat, which is the fat stored around organs. Visceral fat is metabolically active and is known to secrete pro-inflammatory cytokines. By reducing visceral fat, the carnivore diet helps lower inflammation in the body.

Hormonal Balance and the Role of Fats

Next, let's touch upon the equally important issue of hormonal balance. Look upon dietary fat as a kind of lubricant that keeps the machinery inside you running smoothly. First of all, fat is not only fuel; it is structurally incorporated in the making and maintenance of hormones themselves. Sex Hormones Dietary fat allows for the synthesizing of sex hormones such as estrogen and testosterone. These hormones are crucial not only for their general roles in the reproductive system but also because they affect mood and overall good health. Diets that are extremely low in fat can upset this critical balance and lead to problems such as irregular periods, low drive, and even depression.

Just like the adrenal glands, thyroid function depends upon fat for optimum functioning. It regulates body metabolism and energy levels. Fats are required for making thyroid hormones, which, in turn, influence many metabolic functions. Low-fat diets can impede thyroid functions, causing symptoms such as fatigue, weight gain, and cold intolerance. Studies have shown that moderate intake of healthy fats maintains hormonal balance in the body and prevents hormonal imbalances caused by excessively low-fat diets. In dieting, fats are the masked heroes that maintain hormonal systems at optimal function and balance.

Zajac Study and Ketogenic Diet in Athletes

Now, let me put it all into perspective, which led to a study by Zajac (2014)[3]. The main objective of that

---

[3]Zajac A, Poprzecki S, Maszczyk A, Czuba M, Michalczyk M, Zydek G. The Effects of a Ketogenic Diet on Exercise Metabolism and Physical Performance in

research was to see the effects of a ketogenic diet (rich in polyunsaturated fatty acids) in the long run-on exercise metabolism and aerobic performance in off-road cyclists. They also wanted to see the effects of a ketogenic diet on body mass and body composition. The research was conducted on eight male subjects between the ages of 25 and 31. All the participants had a minimum of five years of training experience and participated in off-road cycling.

The above-mentioned study found that a ketogenic diet in athletes led to positive changes in their body composition and lipid levels. It also resulted in **improved oxygen uptake during exercise, which was likely due to reduced body and fat mass. The cyclists also showcased increased fat oxidation.** Heart rate and oxygen intake were higher at rest and during low-intensity exercise. However, they were significantly lower during high-intensity exercise. Additionally, muscle damage during and after exercise decreased after following the ketogenic diet.

This study is a perfect example of how embracing healthy fats may just be the way to go. It also highlights the importance of questioning what we have learned to believe about diet and appreciating the value of fats in

Off-Road Cyclists. Nutrients. 2014; 6(7):2493-2508. https://doi.org/10.3390/nu6072493.

their entirety in our health and performance. As we conclude our studies on the ketogenic state and balance of hormones, remember that your choice of fuel—glucose or fat—can significantly impact the quality of your life. Adopting a balanced approach toward dietary fats as a secret to the full realization of your body's potential may be important in all this.

With that, Fat isn't just back on the menu—it's taking center stage in the performance of your life. It is time to embrace this long-lost metabolic hero and let it fuel your journey toward optimal health. I encourage you to experiment with a balanced approach to dietary fats (saturated, monounsaturated, and omega-3-rich fats) and reflect on how they feel physically and mentally after making the switch. So, tell me, who's ready to become friends with fats again?

Citations of key recent studies and trials that have examined the relationship between dietary fats, heart disease, and overall health, including PREDIMED and PURE trials:

1.PREDIMED (Prevención con Dieta Mediterránea) Trial

- o Estruch, R., Ros, E., Salas-Salvadó, J., Covas, M. I., Corella, D., Arós, F., Gómez-Gracia, E., Ruiz-Gutiérrez, V., Fiol, M., Lapetra, J., Lamuela-Raventós, R. M., Serra-Majem, L., Pintó, X.,

Basora, J., Muñoz, M. A., Sorlí, J. V., Martínez, J. A., & Martínez-González, M. A. (2013). *Primary Prevention of Cardiovascular Disease with a Mediterranean Diet.* New England Journal of Medicine, 368(14), 1279-1290. DOI: 10.1056/NEJMoa1200303

This landmark study showed that a Mediterranean diet rich in healthy fats like olive oil and nuts significantly reduced the risk of major cardiovascular events in high-risk individuals.

2. PURE (Prospective Urban Rural Epidemiology) Study

o Dehghan, M., Mente, A., Zhang, X., Swaminathan, S., Li, W., Mohan, V., Iqbal, R., Kumar, R., Wentzel-Viljoen, E., Rosengren, A., & Teo, K. (2017). Associations of fats and carbohydrate intake with cardiovascular disease and mortality in 18 countries from five continents (PURE): a prospective cohort study. The Lancet, 390(10107), 2050-2062. DOI: 10.1016/S0140-6736(17)322523

The PURE study provided compelling evidence that higher fat intake, including saturated fats, was associated with a lower risk of mortality, while higher carbohydrate intake was associated with a higher risk of mortality, challenging conventional dietary guidelines.

3. Meta-Analysis on Saturated Fats and Cardiovascular Disease

- o Siri-Tarino, P. W., Sun, Q., Hu, F. B., & Krauss, R. M. (2010). Meta-analysis of prospective cohort studies evaluating the association of saturated fat with cardiovascular disease. American Journal of Clinical Nutrition, 91(3), 535-546. DOI: 10.3945/ajcn.2009.27725

This meta-analysis found no significant association between saturated fat intake and the risk of coronary heart disease, stroke, or cardiovascular disease, questioning the long-standing recommendation to reduce saturated fat intake.

These studies highlight the evolving understanding of fats, particularly their role in cardiovascular health, and challenge older paradigms that demonize all forms of dietary fat.

Chapter 5: Carbs: The Ex You Can't Seem to Quit

We've all had that one ex we couldn't quite get over—no matter how toxic the relationship was, something kept pulling us back. Carbohydrates are that ex in your diet. Their allure is irresistible, sweet, and comforting, giving you a temporary high, but the crash that follows leaves you in worse shape than before. The truth is, it's time to let them go.

The Roller Coaster of Carbohydrates

Just like stepping onto a thrilling roller coaster, consuming refined carbs and sugars launches you on an exhilarating high. Once digested, carbohydrates release glucose into the bloodstream, spiking your energy. Dopamine floods your brain, giving you a rush that feels like a bungee jump. But soon, insulin kicks in, sweeping that glucose into your cells for energy use. That's when the crash happens, leaving you exhausted and craving more sugar to feel alive again. This ride never stops—until you decide to get off.

When your body receives more carbs than it can burn, excess glucose is stored in the liver, muscles, and eventually as body fat. This roller-coaster of highs and crashes leads to overconsumption, weight gain, and, ultimately, long-term damage like insulin resistance, where your cells stop responding to insulin's efforts to control blood sugar. The result? A pathway straight to obesity, type 2 diabetes, and other chronic diseases.

You are now riding the rollercoaster of peaks and troughs that characterize carbohydrate addiction, aka *The Ex.*

How We Got Here

Let's step back in time to get a handle on our relationship with carbohydrates. Imagine our ancestors foraging for sustenance. Berries or honey were rare delights saved for special occasions. The thrill of finding a stash of berries was just like hitting the jackpot, similar to a burst of joy that would keep spirits going high for days. These natural sugars were a thrilling treat, fueling energy in times of scarcity. Now fast-forward to today, where grocery store aisles stretch out like neon-lit streets filled with brightly colored boxes of cereals, pastries, and sugary snacks.

Can you imagine the amazement of a Paleolithic human staring wide-eyed and slack-jawed at shelves stacked high with sugary cereals? Simply put, the sheer quantity would be astounding enough to be a jarring contrast to the scarcity that marked their diet. What was once a special treat is now a crutch, a staple that has propelled a basic shift in our relationships with food and our bodies. Paleolithic humans came across fruits and berries occasionally, whereas modern humans have full access to them 365 days a year—that too, a huge variety to choose from.

Another major difference is that Paleolithic humans ate foods directly from their natural source, either immediately or relatively quickly, before the food spoiled. Modern humans now use chemicals as fertilizers and genetic modifications to dissuade insects and ensure a much longer "expiration" to last through transportation and increase shelf life in grocery stores. Our ancestors would be astounded by the abundance—and likely horrified by its consequences.

Meet Insulin: The Body's Bouncer

As we continue to explain this phenomenon, let's meet the body's bouncer: insulin. It is the welcome committee at a nightclub deciding who gets let into the special party of our cells. When you digest those carbohydrates, especially refined sugars, the insulin goes through the roof. It then opens the gates so glucose can pour in. Of course, if the entrance is pounded by too many visitors— too much sugar—all cells start saying no to entry. They become resistant, like a bouncer who has seen one too many troublemakers and decides to crank up the tension in the ropes. Insulin resistance creates a backlog of glucose in the bloodstream, raising blood sugar levels and contributing to health issues like type 2 diabetes, obesity, and metabolic syndrome, to name a few. The once-reliable bouncer is now overwhelmed, trying to keep the rabble in order, and the party inside turns chaotic.

Using our roller coaster metaphor, this ride never really stops. That high in carbs is appealing, but the constant need for a fix creates a vicious cycle. As our bodies begin to adapt to the higher sugar levels, what once was exciting now needs to be pumped into us at increasingly larger doses to experience the same thrills. The more refined carbs we take in, the more our brains and bodies crave them, and thus, we continue this roller coaster ride of highs and lows.

With this new world comes the necessity to understand the biology of carbohydrate addiction. Through millions of years of evolution, our finely-tuned bodies have been designed for moderation but now suffer under the relentless onslaught of sweet temptation that threatens to derail our health end.

When we disembark from the roller coaster, draw a few breaths and feel the energy drain. However, we would never have to feel this way again if we built a better relationship with the carbohydrate world through the knowledge of our biology, admission of our cravings, and conscious decision-making of balance over the sugar tide.

Carb Confessions: Real Stories of Addiction

In a world where the sweet allure of carbohydrates often leads us down a treacherous path, some users online "came clean" and shared their "Carb Confessions." These submissions hint at the real struggles of people from various health backgrounds.

It's not just science—real people have shared their struggles with carb addiction. From midnight binges to soaring sugar consumption, these stories show how deeply this addiction can take hold. Yet they also prove that breaking free is possible, and the rewards are immense: weight loss, normalized blood sugar, and relief from joint pain and fatigue. These are stories of hope.

Confession 1

"During a stressful week, I told myself that a little chocolate wouldn't hurt.

That little piece usually turned into a king-size bar, then ice cream, and before I knew it, I had polished off the whole tub. I felt like I had betrayed myself at the moment, yet I was staring down the same temptation the next day.

"I was at 350- 400 grams per day of sugar. Quitting was the hardest thing I have ever done, but I'm so thankful I quit almost two years ago. I, too, had massive weight loss, and all blood work and blood pressure magically went back to normal ranges. My biggest surprise was to discover the connection between arthritis and sugar. No more stiff joints for me!"

Confession 2

"I went to bed at 1 AM, convinced I needed a 'healthy' snack. I tiptoed to the kitchen, but one granola bite turned into a full-blown binge. Before I knew it, I was sitting on the floor, surrounded by empty cereal boxes. The worst part? I had to clean it up before my partner found out.

"I stopped all sugar, vegetable oils, and alcohol eight months ago, focused on 75% carnivore, 4 to 6 eggs a day, beef, salmon, chicken, and some pickled veg here and there for flavor. Heavy cream, butter, and tallow became staples, and I lost 12kg with no more gout or joint pain. Better mental clarity and mood. Those "reward" foods are KILLING you, folks, literally. Just eat real food! It makes going out for food challenging but worth it."

Confession 3

"I remember eating a ton of sugar through cereal, candy, pastry, and pretty much everything that had added sugar in it back when I was a kid. Didn't have any problems until I was 17, and started having bleeding gums, lethargy, joint pain, low cognitive function, dry corners of the mouth, etc. Discovered fasting, and it was a total game-changer. I still have my pastry here and there, but my awareness doesn't allow me to overdo it."

These confessions remind us that the fight with carb addiction is very real and relevant.

Carbs' Criminal Record

If Carbs (especially processed carbs) had a criminal record, it would be one hell of a long rap sheet filled with some serious offenses against our health. High-carb diets, especially those rich in refined sugars, are linked to a long list of health issues like Obesity. Excess sugar contributes to weight gain from calories that build up when the body fails to burn fats effectively with insulin resistance. High-carb diets, especially those heavy in processed and refined sugars, are linked to a long list of health offenses, including obesity, type 2 diabetes, cancer, and heart disease. Sugars sneak into foods marketed as "healthy" all the time—whether it's breakfast cereals, yogurt, or even sauces and snack bars.

Type 2 Diabetes is another serious issue. Failure of the body to regulate blood sugar results in this chronic disease over time, overburdening the pancreas. There have also been some associations of high sugar diets with cancers, such as breast and colorectal.

Excessive consumption of carbohydrates, mainly processed carbohydrates, increases triglycerides while decreasing good cholesterol that aids heart health. This leads to increased chances of heart disease. This rap sheet paints a bleak picture of how indulging in carbs can come at a heavy cost.

Whenever you walk through a grocery store, try to catch some sneaky carbs that aren't labeled correctly. Let's walk through the aisles, drawing attention to hidden sugar sources in foods you might think are healthy.

Aisle 1: Breakfast Cereals

Even those that claim to contain whole grains can be full of sugar. Ingredients such as "honey," "corn syrup," or "agave nectar"—just code words for sugar, often masquerading as healthful.

Aisle 2: Yogurts

Yogurts claiming to be low in fat or fruit-flavored may contain just as much sugar as desserts. Always read the label; what looks like an innocent cup has more than 20 grams of sugar.

Aisle 3: Sauces and Dressings

They can also contain sugar—cheesy sauce, ketchup, BBQ sauce, and salad dressings. One tablespoon may contain a rather substantial amount of carbs that unsuspectingly intensify a seemingly healthy meal into a sugar bomb.

Aisle 4: Snack Bars

Marked as healthy, bars are packed with hidden sugars masquerading under the name of "natural sweeteners." Watch out because even "protein" or "energy" bars may have more sugar than a candy bar.

Aisle 5: Bacon and Meats

Yes, I said bacon and meats! These are both absolute carnivore favorites, but you need to be very careful of the sneaky marketing. Marketers know that sugar tastes great, so what do you think they add to bacon? Yes, Sugar, Brown Sugar, Maple Syrup, Honey, Molasses, Cane Sugar, and Agave Syrup. Look for bacon without these ingredients— often uncured. As far as meats are concerned, look for the most naturally raised available foods, such as free-range and grass-fed. Corn feed meat may be genetically modified, and chicken and cattle can be given hormones to grow larger and faster, which may not be ideal for your body.

As we make our way through this supermarket of illusions, the message is simple: education is liberation. So, knowledge about those discreet fiends of carbs tied to healthy choices is an exercise in liberation from addiction. Carb addiction can feel like this endless fight, confessing the temptation and then regret. The underlying issues are there for you to see. Taking a closer eye on what is going into our mouths and learning the steps to navigate all our food surroundings can be where we start on the road to reclaim our health. Of course, this journey toward balance is no easy task, but with each step, we move closer to the complexities surrounding our relationship with carbohydrates.

Carb Withdrawal Survival Guide

You can overcome the feeling of threats when coming off carb addiction with the right tools and strategies for withdrawal. Breaking up with carbs isn't easy, but it's worth it. Here's how you can manage carb withdrawal and transition to a healthier way of eating. It is full of practical tips, meal plans, and coping strategies to help you navigate this journey.

1. Cold Turkey Elimination over Gradual Reduction

Instead of gradually getting rid of all carbs, get rid of them. This will help control the severity of withdrawal.

2. Focus on Whole Foods

Focus on whole, unprocessed foods such as lean proteins, healthy fats, and no-carb. These will feed your body without spiking blood sugar.

3. Meal Planning

Create a meal plan for an entire week—no impulse eating. More importantly, drink a lot of water. Many times, people mistake thirst for hunger.

4. Supplements for Support

Some supplements can actually decrease cravings, balance blood sugar, and improve overall health. One product in particular is the electrolyte drink mix "LMNT," which consists of 1000 mg of Sodium, 200 mg of Potassium, and 60 mg of Magnesium. LMNT provides the necessary electrolytes behind energy production in our cells, nerves, and muscles.

5. Manage Cravings

Learn to recognize when you have a craving but do not act on it. Instead, regulate it with mindfulness and meditation. Exercise also helps reduce cravings and enhances mood. So, put on your running or walking shoes and get some miles in.

Tom's Story: From Diagnosis to Freedom

You might think these measures are drastic, but those who followed through with it swear by it. Much like mine, Tom's life story reflects upon the miraculous change through diet change. He, too, was diagnosed with type 2 diabetes when he was still in his early 40s, and he was very shocked to find himself on this earth with such a reality that he never expected it to be.

At first, he tried to get hold of his disease condition through pharmacotherapy and conventional advice about diet. However, high-carb meals left him feeling unhealthier.

The diagnosis served as something of a wake-up call. Tom was angry and scared. He recognized he needed to do something given the family history of diabetes. He proceeded to institute some of the classical prescriptive advice on diet, incorporating whole grains, fruits, and low-fat foodstuffs. Yet blood sugars just continued to rise.

One night, after a rather dejected visit to the doctor's office, Tom chanced upon this documentary discussing the carnivore diet. He liked that it was uncomplicated, and people had reversed their diabetes. *What did I have to lose?'* he thought. Tom, on his part, started by eliminating all plant-based foods from the diet, leaving only meat, fish, eggs, and some dairy. It was not easy, of course. His system suffered from withdrawal symptoms and cravings characteristic of carb detox. However, he kept going and always repeated his mantra: Get health back.

Within a matter of two or three months, Tom was enjoying miraculous changes. Energy settled, and the desire for sugar and carbs dramatically dissipated. With each week that went by, he felt more empowered and in control of his choices.

It was challenging for Tom to cope with the carnivore diet. Socializing complicated it, especially at parties. People kept asking him what his diet consisted of. But Tom found out that planning would help in overcoming this. He would carry his meals either when going to a party or before a party so he wouldn't be left out.

Tom also began tracking his blood sugar count frequently. He noticed these numbers were dropping gradually. In the following follow-ups, the doctor was amazed at the results, and Tom could see a glimmer of hope for the first time ever.

A year after the diet, Tom's blood sugar was normal, and he was no longer diabetic. The rescue was overwhelming because he felt freed from the bondage of carbohydrate addiction that once held him captive.

Tom's journey, however, was about much more than the food; it was rediscovering his existence. He eventually learned how to cook, with the extensive array of meats he was able to try, and how to share experiences with those who sought him out to learn. Tom is an inspiring case study of huge potential—where diet modification can just flip all issues created by carb dependency. As one person's experience is different, so can another's possibility. Techniques or steps suggested in the Carb Withdrawal Survival Guide can be the way out for those seeking to be free.

You can rewrite your story, too, by recognizing the power carbs have over your health and choosing to take control. Take this journey, rely on support, and remember: change is possible, step by step. It's time to swipe left on carbs and embrace a healthier, more sustainable lifestyle.

Who's ready to make the break?

Chapter 6: Your Carnivore Compass: Navigating Your 90-day Transformation

Embarking on a carnivore diet is like setting sail for a new world. It's exciting, a little scary, and you're not entirely sure what you'll find. But don't worry—I'm your trusty carnivore captain, and I've got the map to guide you through these uncharted waters. Like all great adventures, this one needs proper planning and preparation. So far, I've given you the basics, but now it's time to dive into the details. Let's start with a checklist of essential items you'll need to make this journey smoother.

1. Protein Sources

High-quality protein is your fuel, so make sure you're stocked with the best. This means:

- **Beef**: Ribeye, sirloin, ground beef.

- **Pork**: Belly, chops.

- **Chicken**: Thighs, wings.

- **Fish**: Salmon, sardines.

- **Organ Meats**: Liver, heart.

When possible, choose **grass-fed** beef and **pasture-raised** pork and poultry over grain-fed or caged alternatives.

2. Cooking Gear

Proper tools make a world of difference. Invest in:

- **Cast Iron Skillet or Grill**

- **Stainless steel pans**

- **Slow Cooker, Instant Pot, or Air Fryer**

- **Meat Thermometer**

- **Sharp Knives and Cutting Board**

These tools will make your cooking easier and more enjoyable.

3. Flavor Enhancers

This is essential if you are used to classic American favorites and the intense flavors of processed foods. These flavor enhancers might not replace the taste of junk food, but they will enhance the flavor of your carnivore diet. These enhancers will help bridge the gap:

- **Sea Salt** (Redmond's, Celtic, or Pink Himalayan)

- **Animal Fats** (Butter, Tallow, Lard)

- **Fresh Herbs** (optional, but great for variety)

Remember, butter is back and good for you!

4. Snacks

Carb snacking is never recommended, but if you need to get into the habit of healthy eating and want some snack options to replace the highly processed ones you are accustomed to, reach for:

- **Jerky** (without additives)

- **Pork Rinds**

- **Hard-boiled Eggs**

- **Pemmican** (Pemmican is a mixture of tallow, dried meat, and sometimes dried berries.)

There are now healthy snack options available to carnivores, such as "Paleovalley Beef Sticks," which are made with nutrient-dense, all-natural, whole foods. One amazing snack is homemade bacon bites. You can prepare batches in advance by cutting the bacon into half or quarter portions and then either pan or air fry them.

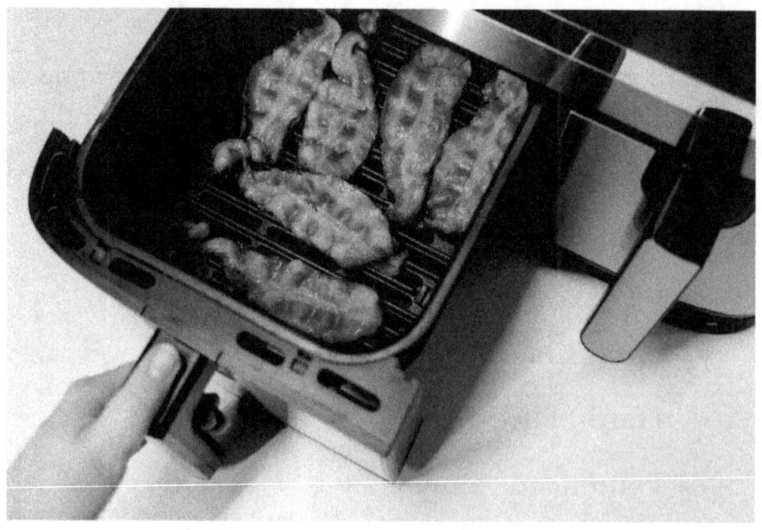

5. Tools for Tracking Progress

Staying on track means keeping a close eye on your progress. Consider:

- A **diary** or **app** to track your meals, energy, and mood.

- A **full blood test** before you start the diet so you can compare your progress over time.

- Carnivore Cookbooks and meal prep guides

The "Do Not Carry" List

Now, let's talk about what to leave behind. Remember that this is an animal-based food diet. The carnivore diet is an elimination diet. You eliminate all the food products that may cause inflammation in the body and instead rely on a natural, animal-based diet.

1. Processed Foods

Say goodbye to:

- Grains (bread, pasta, rice)

- Sugars (sweets, desserts)

- Junk or processed snacks

2. Fruits and Vegetables

While it may seem counterintuitive, **fruits** are high in sugar, and many **vegetables** contain irritants that could impact digestion and inflammation. For the best results, eliminate these as well.

3. Negative Mental Attitude

None of this preparation will matter if you don't believe in your ability to succeed. A positive mindset is crucial for seeing this through. You might feel some initial resistance—this is natural. With the right mindset, you'll push through.

The First Week: Boot Camp

The first week of your carnivore adventure will be the toughest but most important. Think of it as a **boot camp**—a crash course in adapting to this new way of eating. Carnivore diet boot camp can be a great way to dip your feet into this world. Think of it as a one-week life-changing experience. Prepare well, be sharp during the boot camp phase, and maintain a log as a testimony of your journey. Whenever you try something new, your body and mind show some resistance. This is basic Newton's physics: the law of inertia. This is what to watch out for:

In the first week of body boot camp, you will start to adjust in little ways, and your system will begin to learn this new eating pattern. Here's what might be going on in your body to watch for:

1. Carnivore Flu

The symptoms include fatigue, headache, irritability, cravings, and changes in digestion. You can reduce these symptoms by keeping your body hydrated and replenishing electrolytes such as LMNT. Improve fat intake gradually to gain energy level and rest well; engage in light exercise for relief.

2. Energy Level

You will probably feel pretty lethargic in the first week, but by around the tenth day, you will likely start to notice energy coming back. Capture your energy levels every day in your Captain's Log to see the gradual increase, and don't get discouraged by the initial decrease.

3. Sleep Quality

Some sleep better at first, and some are interrupted in the beginning. Maintain your routine and sleep at approximately the same time each night, and create a relaxing pre-sleep routine.

4. Digestive Changes

Bowel habits will change, but it's perfectly okay. Pay attention to the signals from your body and eat enough fat for digestion. You will notice less bloating and gas. Expect fewer bulky stools mainly because your body absorbs more of the natural product, and there is no excess bulk or fiber or man-made chemicals to remove. Remind yourself of the purpose and the intent of why you decided to go down this path.

Tracking Your Progress: The Carnivore Captain's Log

To monitor your progress and make necessary changes, make sure you make your own "Carnivore Captain's Log." Take a diary every week to record the following

1. Weight Change: Note weight changes weekly.

2. Energy Levels: Rate from 1-10, noting changes.

3. Sleep Quality: Rate from 1-10 and note patterns.

4. Health Markers: These include mood changes and skin health.

5. Specific goals: This might include muscle gain, fat loss, or weight management.

At the end of every week, reflect on success and challenges. If your goals or your strategy has changed, adjust it, and you'll be excited about your progress again.

Troubleshooting Cravings and Challenges

There will be days when your body has a mind of its own, especially in the beginning. On these tough days, remind yourself why you started. This isn't about immediate pleasure—it's about long-term health.

To undertake a diet based on carnivores is, to some extent, venturing on a big adventure: some exciting discoveries are possible, but it also poses a good number of potential challenges. All the promised success requires a clear plan and an appropriate mindset.

Consider that every week of the first month you are on the carnivore diet is another destination, different in its challenges, tips, and milestones that will make you adjust to this change—from familiarizing yourself with the basic concepts to exploring diverse dietary options and overcoming obstacles. Together, with guidance from the community and self-reflection, you will be well-endowed with confidence to sail through your carnivore journey, where the 'discovery' would include not only new tastes but the real discovery about your body and your health.

But we all know life is never a walk in the park. There might be days when your body has a mind of its own, and you feel intense cravings—especially in the beginning. For that, think of the carnivore diet journey as putting on different hats, each representing a different diet with its benefits. Remember that you are eating for "Health," not "Pleasure."

Think of the carnivore journey as **wearing different hats**. Each "hat" represents a different style of diet tailored to your needs:

- The '**Standard Carnivore Hat**' is a simplistic approach since it involves mainly beef, pork, and poultry, making it very accessible to a starter audience.

- The '**Nose-to-Tail Hat**' is a good choice for anyone wanting to add nutrition through organ meats eaten together with muscle cuts that may provide you with precious quantities of nutrients and elements for healthy living.

- The **Dairy-Inclusive Hat**, for those who tolerate dairy, adds higher-fat dairy like cheese and cream, which may be included for increased flavor and texture.

With these 'hats,' you can experiment and then find the perfect combination according to your tastes, nutritional needs, and lifestyle.

Just because you are restricted to a certain diet doesn't mean it has to be boring. You can keep your meals interesting while having the power to create a long-term eating pattern that works in line with your personal goals.

You can regard your carnivore journey as a series of exciting island-hopping adventures, where each week will present a new chance for growth and self-discovery. Tread through the storm, change tactics, and enjoy the vibrant landscape of the carnivory world.

Community Support: The Carnivore Crew

It's hard to sail solo. The beginning of this carnivore diet may appear to be entering uncharted waters. In that case, the "Carnivore Community" concept needs to be put in place for support. Finding support and sharing the experiences with others can make your journey much more fulfilling as you feel motivation, encouragement, and belongingness. I highly recommend "The Steak and Butter Gang" on YouTube.

Finding local meetups, online forums, or strategies to deal with unsupportive friends and family members can be the lifeline needed to keep moving toward goals.

One effective way to get immersed in a carnivore lifestyle is to associate with people interested in your kind of lifestyle. The local meetups provide the opportunity to meet like-minded individuals. To find such gatherings, try looking on YouTube and Facebook Groups specifically for the carnivore diet. At times, these meetups have potlucks in them, where people share dishes they like to make, and then you bond with food in the process, learning about different recipes and tips.

If meetings are not possible in person, online forums provide a safe space to talk about questions and share information. One place online is the specific subreddit for the carnivore diet on the Reddit website, such as r/carnivore and r/zerocarb. Members share experiences, challenges, and triumphs within these online communities. By joining these forums, you will find it easier not to feel isolated with the journey you have decided to take.

It is impossible to please everyone with your dietary decisions, and that's perfectly okay. It can be tough to live through the resistance from unsupportive friends and family members, but there are constructive ways to deal with this. First, be open about why you decided to go on that diet. Share your goals— whether it's to reduce weight, be healthier, or gain muscle. This way, you can dispel myths and gain sympathy. It is amusing to me that nobody will bat an eye if someone is eating a large chunk of birthday cake covered in thick frosting but look out if you are having a burger with no bun!

It might also be crucial to set some limits. Be polite in refusing when they force you to eat food that does not fit your diet and thank them for their concern. Tell them your choices concern your health and well-being, not a judgment on theirs. In case of disputing conversations, steer them to mutual interest topics or even some activity that does not primarily rely on eating.

Success Stories

Success stories are a compelling motivator inside the Carnivore Community, and many people have started the 90-day carnivore challenge, which has changed their lives for the better, thus inspiring others to take the step into this dietary journey.

For example, Sarah is a mother of two and is 34 years old. She had experienced years of obesity and chronic fatigue. Before going on the carnivore diet, she was stuck in dieting failures and concerned about the way she looked. Three months after starting the diet, she lost 40 pounds and reported having more energy than ever; for this reason, she continued the Carnivore diet and encouraged her family toward it as well. A remarkable transformation can be seen through Sarah's before-and-after photos. She had to say this: "The carnivore diet gave me my life back. I feel vibrant and not sluggish at all like before. Even my kids noticed the difference in my energy."

Josh was another person who had fought his weight his entire life. He says he goes to the gym for two hours five days a week and only lost two pounds during three months. Josh was frustrated at putting in his all, yet he received no return. He tried every diet, but his weight kept increasing and peaked at 420 pounds.

Josh eventually had weight-loss surgery. The operation involved making his stomach much smaller so he would not feel nearly as hungry. He lost some weight at first, but he still weighed around 365 pounds. The extra weight was really hard on his body. Josh reported that he is about five feet six inches tall, and the weight made his joints ache.

He then tried a different approach with intermittent fasting, which led to the ketogenic diet. As Josh described, he experienced some benefits from the ketogenic diet but felt he could do better than that. He heard Jordan Peterson, an advocate of the carnivore diet, on the Joe Rogan podcast after the birth of his daughter. It was a good push for him as he wanted to have the energy to be a good dad to his newborn daughter. Josh researched the carnivore diet and gained knowledge from two physicians, Dr. Shawn Baker and Dr. Ken Berry.

He started a strict all-animal product diet. Other than tweaking his electrolytes, he found that he had no problems switching from keto to following a diet that was simply carnivore. The more he was on the diet, the more energy he had. He started walking several times a week and noted that his walks became longer with time. This was when he claimed the excess fat practically "shredded off." Now, for two years, Josh has been on the carnivore diet and weighs 180 pounds. The joint pain is gone, and the energy is highly improved.

Like many others shared within the community, these stories help demonstrate how thoroughly the carnivore diet can transform a person. It is not just limited to physical changes but, most importantly, to the psychological and emotional accommodations that a person may undergo after committing to this lifestyle. The Carnivore Community is a fundamental component of one's experience in the carnivore diet. Support through local meetups and online forums will greatly improve your journey, making it easier to stay committed and motivated.

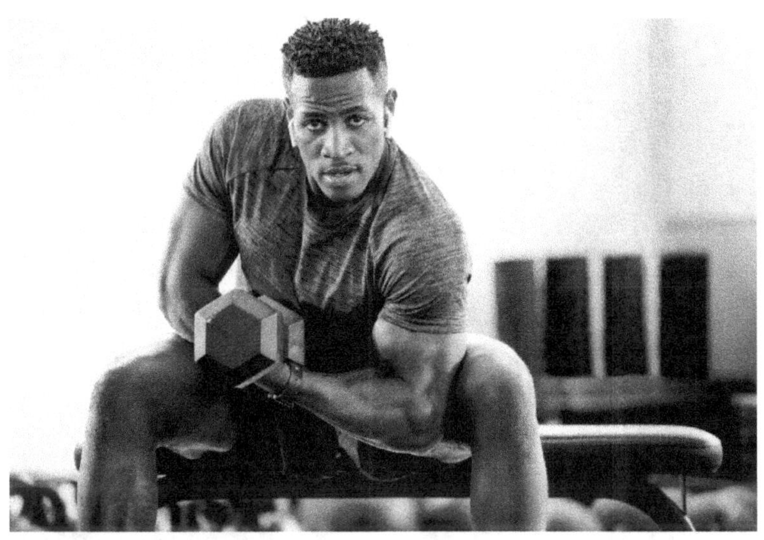

Ready to Set Sail?

With your carnivore compass in hand, you're now ready to chart your course through the first 90 days of your transformation. Remember, you're not alone—the Carnivore Community is right there with you. So, are you ready to set sail on this incredible adventure?

Let's do it—your new, healthier life is waiting just over the horizon!

Chapter 7: The Carnivore Kitchen: From "Meat and Potatoes" to Culinary Mastery

Do you think a carnivore diet means boring meals? All steaks and sausages, right? Think again! We're about to turn your kitchen into a meat lover's paradise that would make even Gordon Ramsay raise an eyebrow in approval.

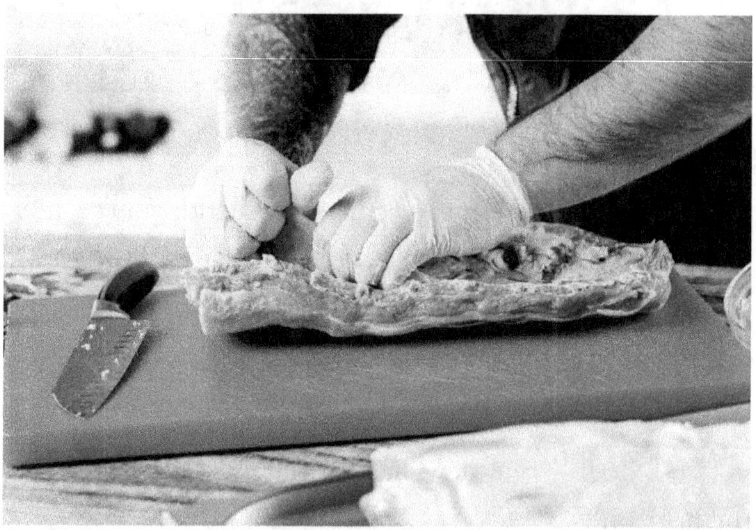

Choosing the Right Meat: The Matchmaking Process

Your carnivore journey begins with picking the perfect protein partner. Various cuts of meat offer different flavors, textures, and preparation methods, allowing ultimate flexibility in your meals. Let's start by breaking down the basics:

- **Beef**: The ribeye brings rich, fatty flavor; sirloin offers leaner options, and brisket provides slow-cooked tenderness. Flanken ribs are an inexpensive wonder meal.

- **Pork**: Opt for pork belly for richness or tenderloin for a leaner alternative.

- **Chicken**: Thighs provide juicy flavor, while breasts are your go-to for lean protein.

- **Fish**: high in omega 3's such as salmon, trout, sardines, and tuna

Grades, like the USDA Prime, Choice, and Select, will determine the quality of the meat; while marbling and tenderness can be part of these characteristics. To truly develop the best flavors and textures when steaks are cooked, experiment with different grades and cuts. Remember that marbling indicates fat, which is beneficial to this diet. During the cooking process, that fat will be rendered down into deliciousness. I used to trim away all excess fat but have now learned that not only does it taste great, but it also embeds a delicious taste into the meat. Don't forget the butter, too! The source where you are acquiring your meat also matters. Go to local farms or butcher shops, focusing more on grass-fed and pasture-raised meats. That way, you ensure that you have the highest protein quality.

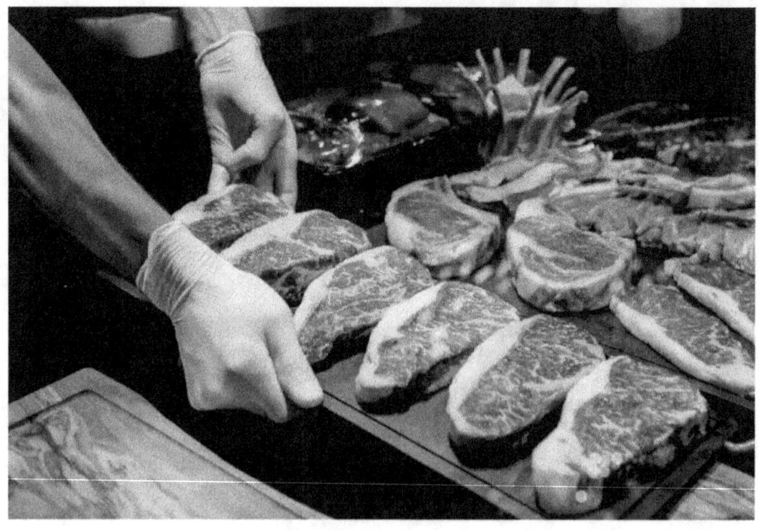

Seasoning Magic: Elevating Your Meat

While the carnivore diet is all about meat, seasoning can take your meals to impeccable heights. Seasoning refers to the art of understanding how various kinds of salts, herbs, and spices can enhance and complement the natural flavors of your meats.

Salt is the most important. Try, for instance, Himalayan pink salt, kosher salt, or sea salt. The more varieties will make every dish unique in flavor and taste. Herbs and spices can vary, too. While some people keep it simple, only with salt, a few other folks might like to add some garlic powder, smoked paprika, or black pepper to spice up their food. The purist carnivore will stick with salt, but you may experiment with various spices to taste and see how they react with your body.

For those who like to experiment, spices like garlic powder, smoked paprika, or even chili flakes can be added in moderation.

Flavor Profile Personality Test

1. Do you like strong and spicy flavors?

- **Yes**: Investigate spices like cayenne, chili powder, or even a hint of smoked paprika.

- **No**: Stick with basic seasonings like salt and pepper.

2. Are you a flavor enthusiast?

- Yes: Try ethnic pastes or spices like gochujang, tika masala, or infused chili oils. Stay away from seed oils; if you want to use oils, the best oil is olive oil.

- No: Only salt shall suffice, but you can try incorporating herbs like rosemary or thyme into your meats to give them a hint of flavor.

3. Do you enjoy rich umami?

- Yes: Add some meat-based umami or fish sauce.

- No: Steer clear of infusion since it's strong on its own.

With the knowledge of meat options and ways to season, you will have the food to fill your belly and arouse your taste buds, making your journey to being a carnivore enjoyable and fulfilling. Remember, the purist carnivore sticks with salt, but feel free to experiment within the bounds of your tolerance.

Mastering Cooking Techniques

When you level up your game and become a deep meat eater, it means your power to master cooking techniques has the chance to become a culinary superpower. I am about to tell you that each of the following techniques adds more flavor to the dishes you prepare while enhancing your cooking experience.

1. Pan-searing: This would be one of the techniques. It involves pan-cooking meat by adding a delicious crust on the outside and sealing the juices inside. Pan-searing is ideal for steaks and pork chops. Pan-searing can be perfected only with the use of a well-seasoned cast iron skillet, allowing the meat to come up to room temperature, and of course, the pan needs to be perfectly hot before introducing the meat into it.

2. Air Frying: This method is a lot cleaner than pan-searing as the grease is contained and captured. Some Air Fryers allow dual cooking elements with separate basket drawers, allowing two dishes to be cooked at the same time.

3. Sous-Vide: Life-changing for those who demand nothing but precision. Essentially, you would seal food in a bag and cook it in a water bath at controlled temperatures for an extended period. It is ideal for cooking meat according to your preference. The cons include specialized equipment to prepare, but the result is melting tenderness and flavor— totally worth the investment.

4. Smoke and Grilling: Smoking will give you one of the richest flavors you can extract from a given cut. Whether grill or stovetop, you can choose the right wood chips— hickory, mesquite, or applewood— for a unique taste. Everyone loves food cooked on an outdoor grill. Slow grilling over hot coals can become a family tradition where people gather around and socialize while the meat slowly cooks to perfection.

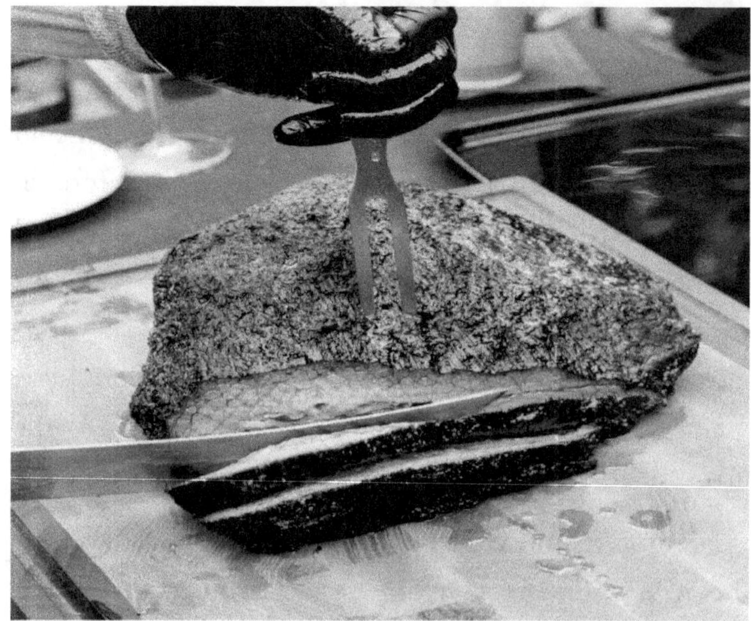

With all these techniques mastered, the inner culinary superhero in you will be unleashed, and those scrumptious meals will consistently impress you and others. Once you get accustomed to these, it's time to bring out the big guns and organ meat.

Exploring Organ Meats: Nature's Multivitamins

Organ meats are often called "Nature's Multivitamins" in the world of eating like a carnivore. These nutrient-rich foods have a series of associated health benefits, and each type contains its special powers.

For example, the liver contains vitamins A and B12 in abundance, which are necessary for synthesizing energy and improving immunity. The heart is rich in CoQ10, keeping the cardiovascular system healthy and supporting energy levels significantly. The kidneys are a highly rich source of iron and essential fatty acids, and bone marrow is full of healthy fats and minerals.

Making organ meats more palatable for beginners can be achieved by blending them with familiar dishes. The ground liver may be mixed into burgers or meatballs, and the kidneys may be included in small quantities in stews where flavors blend together well. Marinating organ meats may also help mask their pungent flavor.

Adding organ meats to your diet brings the remarkable health benefits they offer and acts as an important supplementation in your carnivore journey.

Organ meats are not mandatory, but they provide a nutritional powerhouse. You can always rely on blood tests to monitor your nutrient levels and adjust your intake of organ meats or supplements accordingly.

Condiments and Sauces: Elevating Your Meat

Whereas a superhero always sports signature accessories, the same way, the carnivore diet followers can also augment their dishes with condiments and sauces that give flavor while preserving diet principles. In most cases, condiments are plant-based products; however, you can readily think of tasty homemade versions through creative means. When utilizing condiments, read the labels and stick with those containing natural ingredients. If the ingredient list is long or you can't pronounce the item, put it back down. You can always make your own!

1. Bone Broth: Delicious and so healthy, it's such a great base for soups or just served on its own. You just stew bones with water, salt, and any other allowed seasonings for hours to extract the best flavor.

2. Butter: Elevate your grilled steaks and seafood using a simple butter. Some carnivores may add small amounts of herbs, such as garlic, into their diet. Mashed-up grass-fed butter, minced garlic, and small amounts of fresh herbs [parsley, rosemary, oregano, or thyme] mixed and melted over your cooked favorite meats will give you a great shot of additional flavor. Please note that purist carnivores will only use salt and butter. Your taste buds will adapt, and the meat's natural flavor and textures will replace the old habit of over-seasoning.

3. Carnivore Mayo: Mayo may be homemade with egg yolks, carnivore-friendly oil, salt, and perhaps a touch of mustard to flavor. This condiment adds richness and zest to your dishes but doesn't overdo it. Remember, moderation is key!

Here is the recipe for you to try:

1. 1 large egg (preferably at room temperature)

2. 1 cup of neutral oil (like beef tallow, pork lard, or light olive oil)

3. 1 tablespoon of mustard (optional; use if you want flavor)

4. Salt to taste

4 Mustard: Mustard is typically not considered carnivore-friendly because it usually contains ingredients like vinegar and spices derived from plants. However, some people on a more flexible carnivore diet may choose to use mustard in moderation, particularly if it doesn't contain added sugars or other non-carnivore ingredients. If you're strictly adhering to a carnivore diet, it's best to stick with animal-based seasonings.

With these flavorful options for accessorizing your meat, you will make your food tastier and present an interesting, fulfilling meal within the bounds of your carnivore diet. Try out these cooking techniques, organ meats, and creative condiments to enjoy the journey that is ahead of you.

Creative Carnivore Recipes

Now that you've entered the world of carnivores, you need to go beyond grilling that steak with more scrumptious creative recipes from your protein. Here's a selection of delectable dishes that also represent the true potential of meat so that all your meals remain an exciting and fulfilling experience. Let's start with a classic:

Adapted Shepherd's Pie

Ingredients

- 0.29 pound (130 g) ground or thinly sliced beef or lamb

- 0.04 pound (20 g) smoked slab

- 1 tablespoon cooking fat (tallow, butter, ghee)

- 0.07 pound (30 g) raw bone marrow

- Salt (to taste)

- Pepper (optional)

0.18 pound (80 g) celery root

Method

- Pre-heat the temperature to 220°C and keep the oven on grill function.

- Add the meat and fry it on high heat for a few minutes. No water should be left; if it happens, then fry till all the water evaporates.

- Add the meat to the individual oven dish.

- Peel and chop the celery into small cubicles and cook in water till soft.

- Drain water.

- Add salt and marrow and mix it smoothly.

- Spoon the mash over the meat.

- Bake for about 20-25 minutes, or until golden.

- Enjoy!

Individual portions and baking dishes make this an easy meal for any number of people. Prepare ahead and bake before eating. You can use thinly sliced beef if that is what you have in your house. You can also use ground beef or lamb if you like.

Breakfast Muffins

Ingredients

- 8 ounces ground beef

- 9 large eggs

- 1 teaspoon salt

Instructions

- Preheat the oven to 350F or 175C.

- Grease a standard muffin tin lightly.

- Brown the meat in a skillet over medium heat.

- Whisk the eggs together in a big bowl. Add meat and salt. Stir to combine.

- Distribute the mixture evenly among the muffin tin. Fill well until ¾ full. Bake for 20 minutes or until the eggs are set.

Take it out of the oven and cool for five minutes. Run a knife around the edge of each muffin to release. Pop out onto a wire rack or serve. Serve any leftovers chilled or pop them into the oven and serve. This simple dairy-free breakfast idea is great for meal prep.

Carnivore Stroganoff

Ingredients

- 1 pound ground beef

- 1 teaspoon salt

- 1 cup Beef Bone Broth

- ¼ cup heavy cream

Instructions

- Lightly brown the meat in a skillet over medium-high heat. Use a spatula to break down clumps of the meat if they have formed.

- Add in bone broth and cream.

- Season with salt according to taste.

- Bring to a simmer; cook uncovered for 5 to 10 min and reduce liquid by half.

- Serve hot.

It's a hearty dinner and can be ready in under 30 minutes. What's great about this recipe is that it's flexible, and you can easily modify it for your family to fit their diet, whether keto or another. This classic comfort food is creamy and made purely of animal products.

Meal Prep for Success

Planning ahead makes sticking to the carnivore diet easy. Batch cooking, freezing meals, and investing in quality storage containers will ensure you always have something on hand. Whether it's roasted chicken or steaks prepped for the week, meal prep is your key to success.

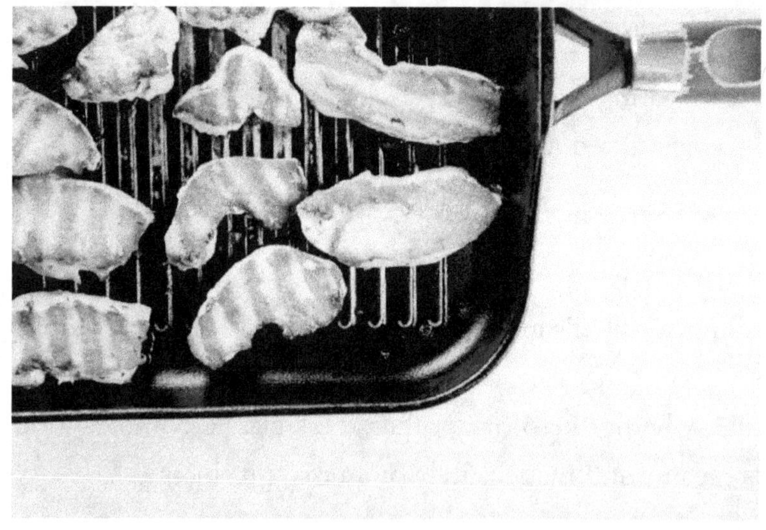

1. **Batch Cooking:** Prepare your meats in large quantities to store, such as roasting multiple chickens or grilling several packs of steaks for that week's meals.

2. **Storage Solutions:** Invest in some quality glass containers for easy reheating. Label what you have for meals and store them in the fridge.

3. **Freezer-friendly:** Focus on preparing easy-to-freeze meat dishes. That would mean making soups or casseroles. Eat it fresh and freeze whatever portions you have left to reheat later.

Most people have trouble with letting go of fast food and cutting out processed food because they are readily available. But with proper meal prep, you can combat that issue. The value of prepping meals pays off with proper planning during the week so that your diet doesn't become a burden for you.

Plating and Presentation

It is possible to make even the simplest dishes more attractive by using a little creativity in presentation. Your 'art of plating' is supposed to make your carnivorous meals attractive; maybe it will even boost your appetite to go out there and show the world your work.

Next time you find yourself in the kitchen, try these tips to trick your brain into thinking you are eating a fancy meal from a top restaurant.

1. Stack your meats creatively or arrange them in a visually pleasing manner on the plate. Use the various sauces to decorate the plate, making it look gourmet.

2. Garnish your dish with herbs, edible flowers, or even slices of lemon. Add color, contrasting shades to your dish, and so on. This makes your food more visually appealing and appetizing.

3. Sharing your plated masterpieces on social media can help build a community and encourage others to understand and appreciate the beauty of a meat-centric diet. With these recipes, meal prep strategies, and plating techniques, you can enjoy and celebrate the flavors of a carnivore diet. Use hashtags like #properhumandiet or #carnivore.

4. Food photography can also help you document and share your culinary journey, building a community and inspiring others along the way.

With these recipes, techniques, and tips, you'll enjoy every bite of your carnivore adventure. Your kitchen is now your playground, and there are no limits to what you can create.

Chapter 8: Beyond the Belly: Unexpected Gifts of Your Carnivore Journey

You might have started this journey to lose weight or improve your health, but there are some unexpected benefits ahead. The carnivore diet is about to give you gifts you never even thought to put on your wish list.

How Meat Fuels Your Brain, the Brain-Gut Connection

Your brain, the mission control for your body, is closely linked to what some call the 'second brain'—your gut. It holds trillions of these microorganisms that play a part in your body's operation. This complex connection represents what is called the brain-gut axis and shows how diet, especially one that is naturally animal-based, deeply impacts mental health.

The gut microbiome and brain are connected through various pathways that include, but are not limited to, vagal pathways, immune responses, and neurotransmitter production. When you're eating a high-fat meat diet, you're arguably cultivating a microbiome that ideally supports clarity of mind and cognitive performance. Research has shown that a diet heavily reliant on animal-source food can offer other great cognitive advantages.

Cognitive functions like focus, memory hold, and problem-solving ability tend to be improved if the brain gets what it requires from quality sources. The three essential nutrients most abundant in meat are omega-3 fatty acids, vitamin B12, and iron[41].

Don't believe me or the research, then try it for yourself. Why not track your own mental performance? See if you notice a sharper focus or clearer thinking after just a few weeks on the carnivore diet, noting any changes in how you focus during tasks, clarity of thought, and ability to solve problems. You might be amazed at the improvement in your cognitive abilities by the end of the challenge.

Mood and emotional well-being are closely related to levels of inflammation in the body. Being rather low in carbs and potentially inflammatory compounds, this diet will reduce inflammation and improve mood. Some research [5] studies have indicated a connection between high-inflammatory diets and mental health disorders, such

---

[41] Leroy F, Smith NW, Adesogan AT, Beal T, Iannotti L, Moughan PJ, Mann N. The role of meat in the human diet: evolutionary aspects and nutritional value. Anim Front. 2023 Apr 15;13(2):11-18. doi: 10.1093/af/vfac093. PMID: 37073319; PMCID: PMC10105836.
[5]2 Firth J, Veronese N, Cotter J, Shivappa N, Hebert JR, Ee C, Smith L, Stubbs B, Jackson SE, Sarris J. What Is the Role of Dietary Inflammation in Severe Mental Illness? A Review of Observational and Experimental Findings. Front Psychiatry. 2019 May 15;10:350. doi: 10.3389/fpsyt.2019.00350. PMID: 31156486; PMCID: PMC6529779.

as anxiety and depression. A diet high in meat can clear the mental fog and the emotional balance; with lessened inflammation, many find that they feel more energetic and less temperamental. This may testify to the deep impact of food intake on our mental environment.

That's what the brain-gut connection has to say: what you put into your body is connected with how your brain functions. Unlock your cognitive and emotional potential by learning about the advantages of a carnivore diet and the smart choices that come about from within.

Skin Health

But the brain isn't the only place the Carnivore Diet works its magic. Your skin can also benefit in ways you might not expect. One of the most noticeable trends associated with the carnivore diet is its impact on skin health, which has attracted attention regarding health benefits. A decrease in processed foods and relying simply on animal products have been reported to have remarkable improvements in skin conditions, such as acne and elasticity.

Perhaps one of the most visible benefits of going carnivore is how it transforms your skin. Many carnivores have attested that their skin and acne cleared up dramatically. In a place where sugars, dairy, and grains are cut out as common triggers for inflammation and breakouts, people generally find that their skin becomes less reactive. Fan photographs submitted by readers reveal such transformations- from acne-scarring to clearer, smoother overall skin. Check out Steak and Butter Gal (SBG) on YouTube to see her transformation. Some users also note that their skin has become more elastic and, with age, has smoothed out even further. As the diet is high in protein, it also provides building blocks for collagen in the user's body to keep the skin firm and elastic. You can check out some of these results on the subreddits r/carnivore and r/carnivore diet.

Apart from its effect on the skin, a diet that is based on protein will significantly affect the quality of hair and nails. People have coined the effects of this diet as "carnivore glow-up" because following a diet that is full of proteins and essential micronutrients will significantly affect the way you look.

The dominant protein in hair and nails, keratin, is a direct beneficiary of the amino acids found in meat. Micronutrients like zinc, biotin, and iron, commonly associated with red meat, eggs, and fish, promote the healthy growth of hair and enhance nail flexibility.

Many diet followers even report changes in hair and nail strength; they have given stories that say that these become much stronger and less brittle. Positive reviews showed improvements in the thickness, sheen, and luster of hair, as well as increased nail growth and less breakage. In this regard, the carnivore diet is rather unique in enhancing a person's health and aesthetics. The carnivore diet is much more than consumption; it also significantly impacts energy and sleep quality. Many report increased energy and quality of rest as they move away from processed foods and toward nutrient-dense animal products.

Energy and Sleep Quality

To get the full flavor of how the carnivore diet impacts your energy, try "energy mapping." Track your energy throughout the day using a simple 1-10 scale. This is how you can do "Energy Mapping" yourself:

1. **Pre-diet Baseline:** Establish a baseline of your energy for one week.

2. **Day of Diet:** Monitor how you feel throughout the day. Do you now have a lot of energy? Don't you get that midday crash?

3. **Reflection:** Once you have completed recording the length of the diet, compare your energy before starting this diet vs. while on the diet.

Most people report that their energy is much more level and more constant day-to-day while on a carnivore diet. This will probably come from balanced blood sugar as well as nutrient-dense foods.

That's not all. People have reported a positive effect of the carnivore diet on their libido and sexual health. The carnivore diet's benefits are a jolting surprise in that regard. Let's try to keep the conversation tasteful and have a sensitive approach to discussing how changes in diet can result in hormonal shifts that enhance performance and satisfaction.

A diet rich in healthy fats and proteins facilitates the production of various hormones, such as testosterone and estrogen, which play a vital role in sex and behavior. Many followers of this diet report an increase in desire and better performance after adopting the carnivore lifestyle. It is a known fact that the Standard American Diet has high levels of estrogen-mimicking chemicals, which has led to many issues for both women and men. A natural, animal-based diet removes this entirely!

Libido and Sexual Health

Some interesting anecdotes shared by readers include unexpected boosts in confidence and energy during intimate moments—making the carnivore diet more than just a meal plan but perhaps a game-changer for one's romantic life.

Talking about libido is a sensitive topic, but it's worth addressing. Many carnivores report significant improvements in libido and sexual health. It is safe to say that the carnivore diet may generally give a person much more vigor and confidence in oneself, thus leading to an increased interest in sexual activities. Who knew that with this diet, one can improve their dating life and feel more energized for date nights? This can also lead to feeling more comfortable in one's skin and ultimately having a more fulfilling, intimate life.

However, the effects of a carnivore diet are much more vast than just physical changes. A 2023 study by the University of Southern Indiana[6] and the University of Maryland revealed that subjects experienced reduced anxiety and depression when they consumed meat compared to non-meat consumers. Still, it is unclear whether meat eaters possess better mental stability or if people with better mental health tend to eat meat.

However, it is certain that different types of meats, like fish, chicken, and beef, carry nutrients to improve healthy production related to hormones and neurotransmitters that help regulate moods. Such important nutrients include essential amino acids such as tryptophan, vitamin B12, iron, zinc, and omega-3 fatty acids. So, this is one

------

[6] 3 Dobersek U, Teel K, Altmeyer S, Adkins J, Wy G, Peak J. Meat and mental health: A meta-analysis of meat consumption, depression, and anxiety. Crit Rev Food Sci Nutr. 2023;63(19):3556-3573. doi: 10.1080/10408398.2021.1974336. Epub 2021 Oct 6. PMID: 34612096.

possible health benefit of the carnivore diet that has been well-established.

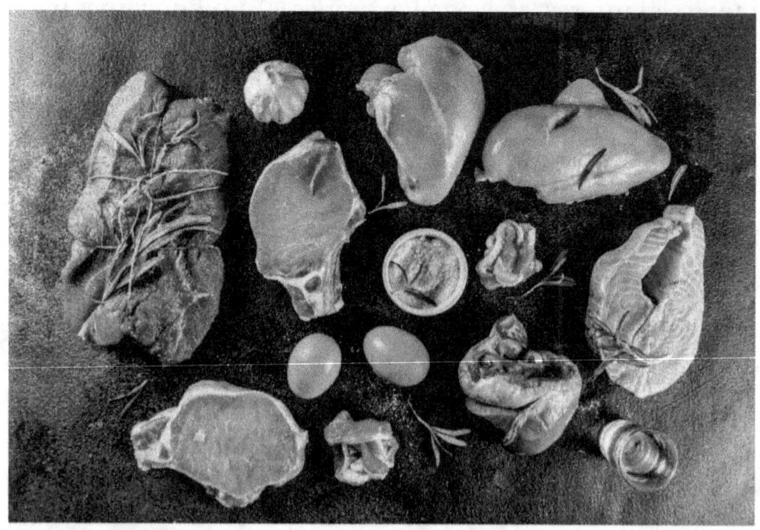

Testimonials

Let's look at some testimonies of people who switched to a carnivore diet as a last resort. On an online forum, Matt reported that all his doctors had been stressing about a low-fat diet after his diabetes diagnosis; therefore, it was surprising for him to find that some people prefer a different approach to managing their blood sugar level.

"I appreciated the concept of potentially reversing my diabetes through natural means. Therefore, I decided to try this unconventional diet and see if it was the key I had been looking for.

"I was initially confused and had many conflicting thoughts about this diet if I am being honest. I was attracted to the probable health benefits that it provided but skeptical about its sustainability in the long term and its inadequacies.

"I knew that the first two or three weeks would be challenging as my body would gradually adapt to extreme changes, but later, I started to like the simplicity of the diet. The food I ate energized my day and was humble yet satisfying. Usually, I had a breakfast of crunchy bacon and scrambled eggs in luscious butter. I indulged myself in succulent beef patties topped with a spoonful of creamy butter for dinner.

"The most challenging and physically demanding time was the first few months. Initially, my body could not cope with this new nutritional profile. I experienced some flu-like symptoms, problems with digestion, fatigue, headache, and confusion in my mind. My low-carb diet began depleting my body's energy, and three months were needed before my system regained its energy.

"The carnivore diet proved to be more than just food—it changed my whole lifestyle, from inside to out. I felt better, lost weight, and saw significant improvement in my overall health."

Who would have thought that giving up on plants might be the door to unforeseen growth in almost everything?

Samuel says everything changed for him. In his words: "In the spring of 2022, I was struggling with low energy, depression, and pain in the joints and back, my pain so strong that I could barely make my way to the office or walk from the car into the movie theater, only to have flare-ups in my knees and ankles for weeks on end. And I walk.

"I also had something called Atrial fibrillation, or AFib. That's an electrical issue affecting your heart's normal sinus rhythm. I knew I needed to lose weight and get healthy—and I needed to do it soon. It is more important now that I can watch my three children grow up to have kids of their own. I wanted to be able to provide for my family.

"But I wasn't sure that would happen with the path I was going down. And that became my biggest motivation. I had heard from some friends who were doing the keto diet and losing weight, so I decided to give that a try. With the keto diet, you limit your carb intake to about 20 grams per day and increase your fat intake.

"I spent the following months studying low-carb diets and watching YouTube videos from doctors and those with experience.

"I had lost very little weight but didn't feel a whole lot different, though. And yet, I kept finding more and more information about the ultimate elimination diet, where you completely cut carbs out of your eating plan. This was the carnivore diet, and in July of 2022, I went full in.

"In that diet, you aren't supposed to eat any of these things; there are no vegetables, fruits, or other carbs. However, I consume beef in great quantities, sometimes eggs and bacon. Chicken wings or chicken thighs sometimes, and pork, too. I don't use any seed oils; I cook either with bacon fat, tallow, or butter.

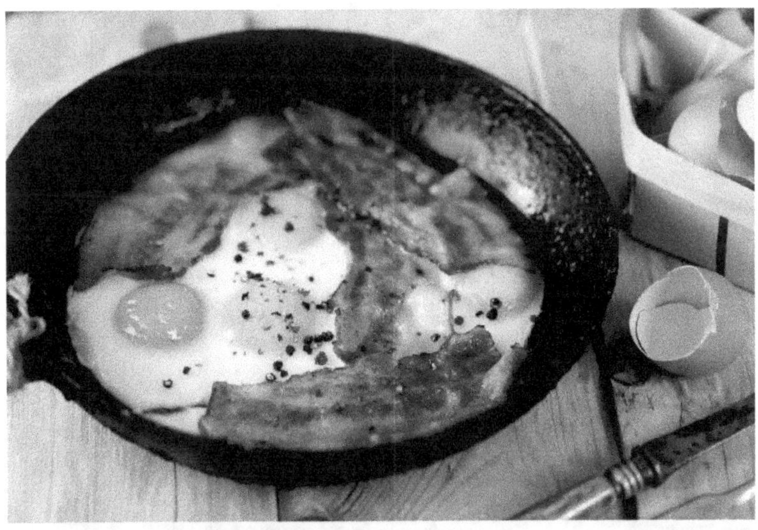

"My typical day of eating consists of a steak around noon, then a couple of beef burger patties-no bun-and either eggs or bacon. I normally eat about two pounds of meat per day.

"I was now down to 65 pounds by early November and had much more energy to do things. What's truly the most amazing thing is that my arthritis and pains from my joints were both gone. I hadn't had a single episode of A-Fib in a couple of months, and I used to get a couple of episodes per week."

With testimonies like this, what's stopping you from trying out this diet? Who knows, eating meat may answer all your health-related concerns.

Chapter 9: The Carnivore Athlete: Crushing PRs on Steak Power

Carb-loading before a big race? That's so last century. Welcome to the era of the meat-powered athlete, where records are crushed on steak, not spaghetti.

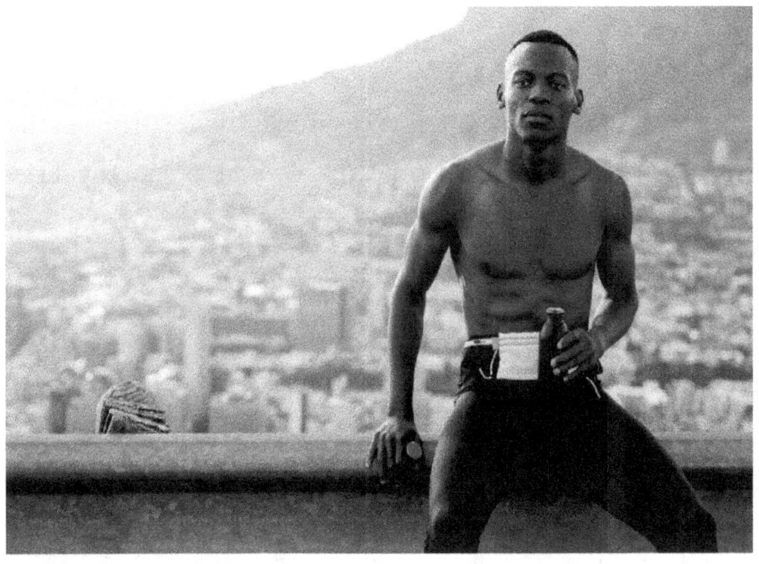

For decades, carb-loading has been the favorite training strategy for endurance events. However, new studies now indicate that this approach may not be as effective after all. Instead, fat adaptation, or the body's adaptation to shift toward a higher use of fat as a fuel source, offers several advantages for endurance performance.

Why Fat Is the Superior Fuel for Endurance

Think of your body's energy stores as fuel tanks. Carbs are like a small, high-octane reserve that burns quickly but runs out fast. In contrast, fat is a massive, slow-burning reservoir. Although the body can hold about 2,000 calories in glycogen, it can hold up to 100,000 calories in fat.

Imagine tapping into this vast resource to support longer durations of activity. By transitioning from carbs to fat as your main fuel, you can avoid the dreaded energy crashes that come with glycogen depletion and instead enjoy sustained, efficient energy throughout endurance events. Let us dissect this topic further for better understanding.

Metabolic Flexibility: The Secret to Peak Performance

The body's ability to efficiently flip between carbs and fats as primary energy sources, depending on what the activity demands, is its metabolic flexibility. High metabolic flexibility in athletes suggests that they can adjust their fuel according to intensity and duration to optimize their performance and recovery.

From the carb-loading myth to an appreciation of fat adaptation, new doors are now open for endurance athletes. Discovering metabolic flexibility using the fuel tank analogy can improve performance and endurance. It is an improvement of energy stores and a means to support health and recovery. Put on your science goggles and let your body run on the fuel it was scientifically designed for!

We all know that the carnivore diet consists primarily of animal products and offers some distinct benefits suited to the specific needs of various athletic activities. To understand this concept adequately, we must learn how this diet can enhance performance in endurance, strength, combat sports, and team sports.

The Carnivore Diet for Athletes: Maximizing Performance

The carnivore diet, with its focus on animal-based products, is uniquely suited to athletes. Whether your sport demands endurance, strength, or agility, this way of eating offers specific benefits that can help optimize performance across various disciplines. Here's how:

1. Increased Fat Burning and Stable Energy

The shift toward fat-burning for endurance athletes allows them to rely on steady, long-lasting energy. With fat as the primary fuel source, they can avoid the energy dips common in carb-dependent athletes, maintaining higher levels of stamina over extended periods.

2. Rapid Recovery and Increased Muscle Mass

Strength athletes need a higher level of protein to be able to repair and rebuild muscle tissue. The carnivore diet delivers this in abundance, aiding recovery and reducing inflammation, which allows athletes to train harder and more frequently.

3. Weight Management and Mental Clarity

Combat sport athletes need either a weight-restricted environment or the possibility of extra energy and clear mental functions to be in top shape. The carnivore diet can help manage weight since it can reduce fat loss without reducing lean muscle mass. It also has anti-inflammatory effects on mental clarity, and athletes can gain a competitive advantage.

4. Reduced Inflammation and Faster Recovery

Team athletes benefit from the anti-inflammatory properties of animal-based foods, which help speed up recovery times and reduce the risk of injury. This is because the higher the number of anti-inflammatory properties they intake through animal-based food consumption, the better chances they have of bouncing back quickly to be trained and compete properly. By incorporating foods rich in omega-3 and other essential nutrients, athletes can recover faster and train more effectively.

Training and Competition Day Nutrition: Fine-tuned for Performance

Tailoring meal plans to match specific sports can yield tremendous benefits on training and competition days. Here are some general guidelines:

Pre-training/Competition: Have a high-protein meal 2-3 hours before activity. Good sources include eggs or lean meat cuts, which are easily digestible.

Post-training/Competition: Recovery is crucial. Focus on the recovery diet through a protein-enriched meal right after the activity. Make sure to incorporate lots of fat for support in recovery and satiety.

Potential Challenges and How to Overcome Them

While the carnivore diet has numerous benefits, athletes should not ignore some possible concerns that may arise from its consumption, including the electrolyte balance. When athletes switch to a low-carb diet with more fats, the body experiences imbalances in sodium, potassium, and magnesium. You can balance this through bone broth and electrolyte supplements.

To help your body adjust and aid in a smoother transition, this is what you can do:

1. **Hydrate**: Hydration is important, especially during the adaptation period. Drink plenty of water and liquids.

2. **Adaptation Periods**: Some athletes face an adaptation period where they can feel weak or sluggish. This is why you should gradually change to the carnivore diet to allow your body to adjust with patience since it adapts itself slowly.

3. **Supplements**: Omega-3s, magnesium, and potassium are your best bets in a healthy supplement regimen. Make sure to incorporate those in your diet.

4. **Electrolyte**: Electrolyte-rich fluids, including bone broth, are key. Add a pinch of salt to your water if you don't have broth on hand to manage sodium. I highly recommend the LMNT product line.

If you are an athlete, the carnivore diet can become a powerful tool for you. Athletes from different disciplines have improved performances through fat burning, recovery, mental clarity, and an inflammation reduction course, all while keeping to a strict animal-based diet. With tailored meal plans and practical strategies aimed at addressing potential concerns, athletes can jump into "precision fueling for peak performance" and then bring out their best.

Fueling the Carnivore Athlete: Pre- and Post-workout Options

While most athletes fuel their workouts with protein shakes and carbohydrate-heavy recovery meals, the carnivore diet offers alternative, meat-based solutions that can be more than inadequate for athletic performance:

Swap out that standard protein shakes with one of these options:

Pre-workout

- **Eggs and Bacon**: This is one of the staple breakfasts filled to the brim with top-of-the-line proteins and healthy fats. The couple will sustain energy without leading to the crash, unlike carbs.

- **Beef Jerky**: This is the perfect snack on the go. It is full of protein and can easily be digested. Beef jerky before you work out is great for quick energy.

- **Bone Broth**: Bone broth, rich in electrolytes and amino acids, can hydrate and feed you before you start working out.

However, following a workout is when recovery meals are needed most. Keeping to a carnivore diet, this is what you can try post-workout or training.

Post-workout

1. **Grilled Steak with Bone Marrow**: This nutrient-dense meal offers protein for muscle repair and fat that will be sustained in the body.
2. **Chicken Thighs with Skin**: It is a high-protein meal with healthy fats for replenishment when you have spent your body's energy.
3. **Pork Belly**: This is a high protein and fat food. With its rich yet satisfying taste, pork belly is one of the best recovery foods for athletes.

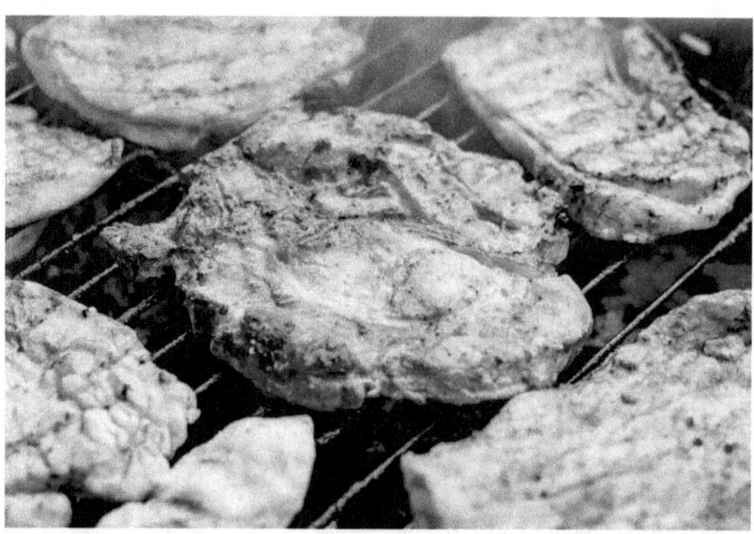

These options not only adhere to the carnivore protocol but also raise the question of whether post-exercise nutrition ever requires refined shakes or carbohydrate-rich foods.

Not just this, a carnivore diet also gives athletes a psychological advantage over their competitors. The psychological edge can be seen on three levels: a stress-reduction level, an emotional/psychological, and lastly, a competitive level.

The Psychological Edge: Mental Clarity and Focus

Most athletes comment on improved mental clarity and reduced anxiety while on a carnivore diet. Reduced inflammation and regulation of blood sugar stabilize mood swings, so they remain sharp and focused more precisely during training and competition.

The nutrient density of animal products supports general brain health, which may help support stress management. In particular, omega-3 fatty acids, which are found in fatty fish, are highly conducive to mood regulation.

As long as you pay attention to the quality of your meals, enjoying every bite can connect you more deeply with your food, make you more satisfied, and bring less stress with eating times. Before competing or working out, you can also visualize your performance. See how you hit movements perfectly, which may bring more clarity and confidence.

Be sure to master deeper breathing patterns to alleviate nervousness and promote greater mental calm. Examples include box breathing, which can be used to help the mind relax before an important competition. With these things in mind, you will outperform yourself and break personal records left and right.

To get a few key insights into how the carnivore diet serves real life, we spoke with a variety of professional athletes from different sports who are now following this diet.

Real-life Success Stories: Athletes Thriving on a Carnivore Diet

1. John, an Endurance Runner

John started on a diet only six months ago and began to experience some very clear differences in his runs at larger distances. He found out he was very reliant on carbs before, but determined to make this work, his body got accustomed to his workouts, and that way, he could maintain a more constant energy level and endurance.

2. Lisa, CrossFit Competitor

Lisa can't get over how much high protein and fat she gets in her meals, and it surely helps her at recovery times. She first began getting some sort of side comments from her fellow athletes, but she has now become an ardent mouthpiece for what she has obtained.

3. Mike, Mixed Martial Artist

According to Mike, he maintains that a diet only of meat allows him to preserve weight and be mentally clearer while fighting. First off was electrolyte management; after that, he used to add bone broth and salt to balance out the whole thing. Once he got used to this routine, he saw himself perform better.

These athletes symbolize how a diet based on meat has aided people in so many different ways—from athletic performance enhancement to more acute mental clarity despite each of their struggles.

The carnivorous diet is a very enticing alternative to the usual pre-and post-workout nutrition systems, and it also provides really creative meat-based options that really fuel performance. Aside from the psychological benefits, especially in terms of enhanced focus and better stress management, the revelations from professional athletes speak of the potential of this approach. By embracing the carnivorous lifestyle, an athlete will unlock physical prowess and a mental edge that separates them from their counterparts in their chosen sports.

The Zach Bitter Example: Record-breaking on Almost No Carbs

Take the example of Zach Bitter. He has become one of the world's ultimate ultra-runners. He recently ran 100 miles in 11 hours, 19 minutes, and 13 seconds at Wisconsin's Six Days in the Dome event last August, which is his latest world record. His time was well over the record set by Russian athlete Oleg Kharitonov at 11 hours, 28 minutes, and 3 seconds.

More amazing, however, is that Bitter trains and competes on almost no carbs. At times, carbs make up as little as 5 percent of his diet, and Bitter claims that even non-endurance record-holders can do the same.

Bitter says he really loads up with animal products, such as salmon, eggs, and red meat if it's a usual day. But if he's doing a big training run, he introduces some carbs again. He feels that "if I'm doing something really strenuous, carbs are an advantage from a training standpoint."

In an interview with Men's Journal, he mentioned:

"In high school and college, I had a whole-food type of approach to nutrition, like a lot of endurance athletes do. At that time, most of the research you'd find was based on a high-carbohydrate diet, so I skewed my nutrition that way. My diet was clean but probably 60% carbs. Then, in 2010, I started participating in ultraendurance events and noticed that things weren't ideal—not being able to sleep consistently through the night, having big energy swings during the day, chronic inflammation in my ankles, things like that."

He was asked when he decided to change his diet, he said:

"Well, I was at a crossroads. One option was to scale back on training, which I didn't necessarily want to do. The other option was to look at what I could do nutritionally, and I made the switch.

"It wasn't like I had this crazy energy drop on the first day. For the first two to four weeks, there were a couple of days when I felt lethargic when I exercised, but I didn't really notice a huge energy deficit when I was just doing routine activities, like walking around or writing on the computer or something like that. Afterward, I felt so much better. The inflammation went away quickly, and within a month, I slept way better, and I felt like I was getting through the night. And I noticed that my energy levels were consistent throughout the day."

With the experiences and knowledge of experts to guide you, take the leap of faith and make the switch. Who knows, maybe you will also find yourself breaking your PRs in no time. The carnivore diet isn't just a way of eating—it's a strategy for peak athletic performance. With the right mindset, a tailored meal plan, and a focus on recovery, athletes of all kinds can tap into the potential of fat adaptation to fuel their training, improve mental clarity, and break personal records. Whether you're an endurance runner, CrossFit competitor, or mixed martial artist, the carnivore diet can be your secret weapon to outperform the competition and reach new heights.

Chapter 10: Raising Little Lions: The Family Guide to Carnivore Living

The health of our children has been rapidly declining in the United States. Diabetes, obesity, early puberty in females, and autism are just some of the ailments impacting our youth. Why is this happening? There may be a strong connection to metabolic health, which is directly impacted by the food we eat.

In today's society, natural food is replaced by highly refined food, stripped, and reformulated into more addictive formulas with man-made chemicals, pesticides, fertilizers, plastics, and preservatives. While the body can process some of these toxins periodically, it cannot cleanse itself from the daily bombardment, let alone decades of poor nutrition intake. What can we do? Teach your children! While it may not be easy to convince children to accept a strict Carnivore lifestyle, it is important to explain the facts of eating in a healthy manner and avoiding processed foods. Any improvement to more natural foods is a step in the right direction.

Imagine your child's lunchbox as the healthiest option in the cafeteria, where they eagerly reach for nutrient-rich bites of energy-packed, delicious food. That's the beauty of carnivore parenting—where 'finish your veggies' is traded for 'savor your steak!

It's surely no small achievement to transition to a carnivorous diet or a low-carb animal-based diet, so it will take some years of patience on your part as a parent. The key is to stay flexible in your approach. The task will undoubtedly be much easier if you have toddlers or primary school-aged children since you generally have a big, if not total, control over what your children eat.

For middle and high schoolers, the shift may be more complex. Their growing independence and social lives can make dietary changes challenging, but flexibility and patience will go a long way.

Regardless, introducing your little ones to the carnivore diet can be a bit daunting. But if you use terms like "superhero training" in the conversation, it just might increase your odds. Encourage them to think of meat as 'hero fuel' that helps build strength, agility, and focus, making it as essential as their favorite cape or gadget.

If worded playfully to describe various types of meat, such as chicken being called "flying fuel," beef as "muscle power," and fish as "brain food," your kids will be more than excited to try this diet out. This makes eating a meat-based diet exciting, turning what may otherwise seem like a daunting transitional period into a fun ride toward becoming their best. Teens will likely respond to autonomy and science. Add in how the Carnivore diet supports both physical and mental endurance, something especially useful for school and extracurricular activities. "Highlight how meat-based meals help stabilize energy levels, sharpen focus, and, for those interested, even aid in strength-building." Since teens are conscious about their appearance and often struggle with body image issues, let them know the effect this diet can have on their bodies. Whether it is gaining muscles or losing weight, a carnivore diet can help them achieve their goal, making it more desirable.

Protein, among other nutrient-rich animal products, provides all vitamins and minerals necessary for cognitive functions and total growth at a time in life when it's needed the most. Testimonials from the parents include improvements in their children's ability to sit still for lessons, accomplish homework more efficiently, and converse more clearly. Telling your kids these success stories may further motivate them to follow this diet and get excited about superhero outcomes.

Parents implementing this strategy with their children have seen a reduction in mood swings at home and improved attention at school; some children even became less hyperactive.

Making the change to a carnivore diet is made more palatable by letting kids plan and prepare. Let them decide what their favorite meats are or help in preparation and frame it like a mission creating 'power-packed meals.'

Challenge them to create superhero names for their dishes, like "Mighty Meatballs" or "Power-up Steaks." Participation such as this will increase ownership and help train them for invaluable skills in the kitchen right from the earliest stage.

You can also put in themed meals or challenges, such as "Carnivore Quest," where points can be gained for trying new types of meat or completing certain meals. The aspect of gamification of this diet can turn a boring diet into a fun activity, and they can see eating meat as part of their superhero journey.

Just because your kids follow a carnivore diet doesn't mean they can't experience tasty flavors and combinations. Here are some kid-friendly recipes you can introduce into your kid's diet to make it fun and nutritious.

Grilled Chicken Strips

- Slice up chicken breasts into uniform strips.

- Lightly season the chicken strips with salt and pepper.

- Preheat the grill.

- Grill the chicken strips on each side for a few minutes until they are fully cooked.

- Optionally, marinate the chicken in lemon juice before grilling it to add flavor.

- Serve the grilled chicken strips with either animal-based dips or on their own.

This is a fun snack which is both healthy and nutritious. This is perfect as an afternoon snack or for their school lunch.

Turkey fireballs

- Preheat the oven to 350°F (175°C).

- Mix ground turkey, salt, and your preferred spices in a bowl together.

- Roll the mixture into small balls about 1.5 inches in diameter and place them on a parchment-lined baking sheet.

- Bake the turkey meatballs for 20-25 minutes or until they are fully cooked.

- You can serve the meatballs or 'fireballs' warm or cold, and for extra flavor, consider adding cheese to the mixture before baking.

Pair the meatballs with either soup or gravy for a balanced meal. This recipe is a wonderful way for your kids to get started on their carnivore journey and get acquainted with various types of meats.

Beef lettuce blankets

- Start by cooking high-quality ground beef over medium-high heat. Break the lumps of meat apart as it browns.

- Season the cooked beef with natural flavorings.

- Spoon the fully cooked beef into large, sturdy lettuce leaves such as romaine or butter lettuce.

- Use the lettuce as a natural wrap to make it easy to hold and eat.

- To keep it kid-friendly, avoid adding spicy ingredients and consider adding some low-carb condiments if your kids enjoy those.

Following these steps will help you create a delicious and nutritious beef lettuce blanket that provides a healthy dose of protein for kids following a carnivore diet.

Raptor Rolls

- Gather high-quality ham slices and pieces of cheese.

- Place a piece of cheese on a ham slice and roll it up.

- Secure the roll with a toothpick to keep it secure.

- You can use different types of cheese for variety, such as cheddar, mozzarella, or gouda.

- Optionally, add a smear of cream cheese inside the roll-up for extra richness.

- Pair the roll-ups with carnivore-friendly sides like cooked bacon or boiled eggs.

- Wrap each roll-up in parchment paper to keep them fresh until lunchtime.

This is another one of those recipes that your kids will love as it includes all their favorite 'junk' items. Kids are simple beings; if they like the look of their food, they will be more inclined to eat it.

For that, you need to give their lunchboxes a makeover to help create school lunches following a carnivore diet. It starts with packing appealing and colorful lunches that are going to get your child excited to eat. Think beyond just plain old slices of meat. Instead, add chicken tenders, beef jerky, or homemade meatballs to the menu. Your child's energy is now coming from fat, so be sure to include natural products with high-fat content.

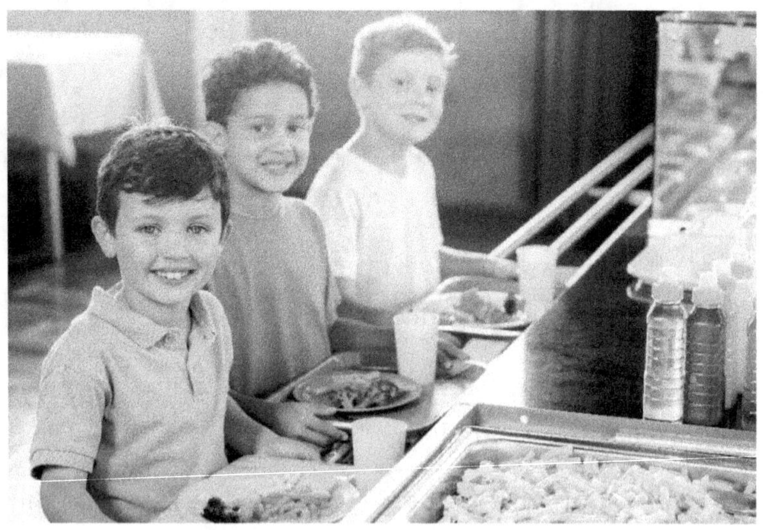

Easy menu items:

- Eggs, hard-boiled or scrambled with cheese

- Bacon snacks

- Bone Broth

- Pork Rinds

- Chicken Thighs. Chicken Wings, Chicken Strips

- Beef Jerky

- Cooked Pork Belly

- Burgers – patties, sliders, healthy tacos mixed into scrambled eggs

- Seafood – fish, shellfish, mollusks

- Fried Chicken Strips

- Cheese, Dairy, and Butter

- Water

Use fun containers that keep the food fresh and appealing, and even add a side of dipping sauce to make it more exciting to eat. Likewise, don't forget to inform school administrators about your child's needs. A brief, friendly email or meeting can help clarify what works best for your child, ensuring they are supported in their food choices during lunch and snack times.

Socialization can become tricky, but a proper plan can help you handle it well. Whenever your child is invited to a birthday party or sleepover, make them understand beforehand the good choices that should be made. You can explain to them the reason behind such choices and the benefits of that.

You may role-play similar scenarios with them and teach them what to do in social situations. You can teach them lines like, "I appreciate the invitation, and I'm following a special diet that keeps me at my best." Simple scripts can also assist parents in explaining children's dietary preferences to other parents. Something like, "We're trying a new approach to eating that is meat centric. Hope that is okay!" is enough to do the trick in most situations.

It will also make your child feel confident when declining non-carnivore options without embarrassment and awkwardness. Leading by example is the way to go to make sure that the carnivore lifestyle turns into a wonderful family experience. Family meals will become something you all look forward to, finally having the opportunity to share pleasant meat-based cuisines.

Engage your children in meal preparation and cooking; they can help choose recipes and prepare different dishes.

This shared responsibility builds their cooking skills, too, and at the same time, strengthens family ties. Put emphasis on the benefits of carnivore meals, such as greater energy. This will lead to fun conversations around the dinner table and normalize the meat-centric diet.

When children see parents enthusiastically embracing the diet, they tend to follow suit. Sincere concern over adequacy issues about nutrients, growth, and social development should not be taken lightly. Pediatric nutrition experts tend to support well-planned meat-based diets in general when they are properly planned, as they help children receive all the nutrients needed. This diet is good and healthy for them, so long as variety is ensured through several cuts of meat and, when appropriate, organ meats that are rich in nutrients can be introduced.

A pediatrician's regular checkups are also necessary to help ensure your child is growing well and getting the right balance of nutrients. From a social point of view, educating kids on how to take control of their food decisions can be a liberating and confidence-building factor for them as they are bound to feel more comfortable in social situations. A balanced perspective will further dispel any anxiety and allow you to support a healthy yet enjoyable lifestyle for the whole family while being a carnivore.

If you have teenagers on a vegetarian or vegan diet because they believe such a diet is healthy and good for the environment, the transition can be daunting.

For older children, you can reason with them (lol), and it is important to engage them in open and non-judgmental conversations about their dietary choices and health implications. Encourage them to explore the reasons for their choices and their potential impact on their well-being. Be supportive and provide them with evidence-based information about the benefits of a carnivore or low-carb animal-based diet. There is so much information available online and on social media such as YouTube that they will be able to access a lot of information very quickly.

If your child is used to a lot of processed food (chips, cookies, candy, crackers, breakfast cereals, soft drinks, sugary drinks, muffins, donuts, french fries, pasta, pizza, frozen meals, etc. etc.), begin by gradually replacing them with healthier homemade alternatives. Your child will be less likely to resist such gradual changes in his diet. Here are a few suggestions:

Prepare High Protein Breakfast: Replace cereal or jam toast with protein-rich breakfasts like bacon and eggs, scrambled eggs, sausages, and egg and cheese pancakes. Ensure that their first meal of the day is high in protein and fat and low in carbs because it will keep your children satiated for a long time and avoid the carb roller-coaster.

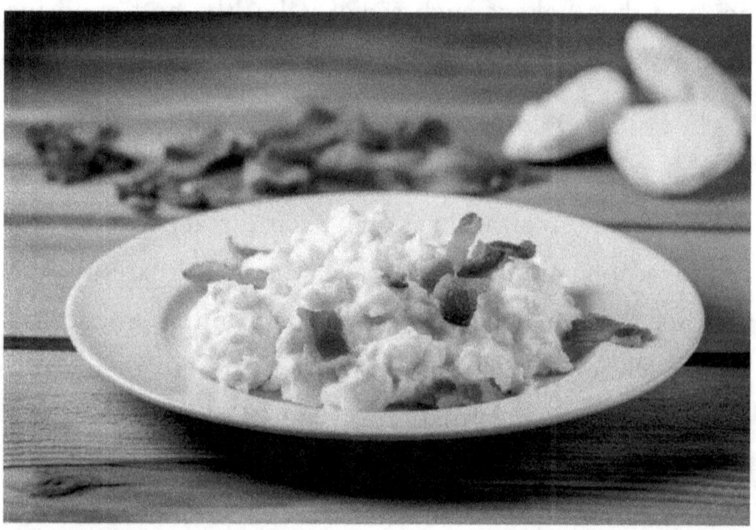

Pack Healthy Lunches for Your Kids to Take to School: If your children are going to school, pack healthy lunches so they do not depend on the canteen foods that are normally high in carbs and not hygienic. Some of the choices include meatballs, burgers without buns, sausages, crust-less quiches made from eggs, minced meat, cheese, and seasonings, sashimi, carnivore fish fingers, boiled eggs, plain whole milk yogurt with chopped fruits, etc. Add healthy, locally sourced vegetables if they want them, but the quality of the meat should be higher than that of any other ingredient.

Replace Sugar-Loaded Fizzy Drinks with Water: Keep water as your primary beverage. Seltzer with no sugar additives is great. These are very tasty, especially when combined with the "Salty" LMNT supplement, giving them needed Sodium, Potassium, and Magnesium. If your children do not have a dairy intolerance, then plain full-cream milk is an acceptable substitute.

Replace Commercial Junk Foods with Better Options: Replace all commercially purchased junk food with natural foods or homemade options like beef jerky, pemmican, pork rinds, yogurt, and carnivore ice cream.

Make Your Sauces and Dressings Homemade: These probably come packed with added sugars and unhealthy fats. Go for versions of homemade ones that involve simple ingredients like bacon grease, cold-pressed olive oil, vinegar, lemon juice, herbs, and spices.

Let me end this chapter with an impressive success story about Mikhaila Peterson Fuller.

https://mikhailapeterson.com/ creator of "The Lion Diet" https://liondiet.com/

Mikhaila suffered from several ailments and an underlying illness as a child, which baffled the medical establishment. She had chronic pain, arthritis, and depression, and much later discovered the underlying illness of Chronic Inflammatory Response Syndrome (CIRS). She was put on medications to ease the symptoms and numb her body. These "treatments" did not address the underlying issue. Through experimentation on her own, she eliminated food sources that triggered her suffering. Mikhaila eventually removed all but steak, salt, and water, which changed her life for the better.

I encourage you to read her whole story, but here is an excerpt from her website: "I cut out any food that I thought could possibly be inflammatory or cause an immune response like an allergy—dairy, legumes, eggs, nuts, seeds, sugar, processed foods. I went down to a diet of greens, some root vegetables like parsnips and sweet potatoes, and meat and fish. Nowadays, this is somewhat similar to a restrictive paleo diet. In a month, my rash healed for the first time since it had begun years prior. Three months later, my fatigue and depression lifted for the first time I could remember in my entire life."

Mikhaila had extreme symptoms and issues that only subsided with a natural carnivore-based diet. Just think of all the benefits healthy children will derive from eating this way and not causing harm to themselves by injecting all the chemicals, preservatives, insecticides, fertilizers, and plastics found in today's highly processed foods.

Chapter 11: The Ethical Carnivore: When Eating Meat Saves the Planet

What if I told you that your steak dinner could be the key to saving the planet? Surprised? It's time to rethink the narrative around meat and sustainability.

I know it sounds odd because we have always been fed the idea that eating vegetables and going vegan is the sustainable option, but that might be a far stretch from the truth. There are various ways in which eating animals can be beneficial for the environment, such as regenerative agriculture. While plant-based diets have their benefits for some people, it's essential to consider the complexities of food systems and the potential for sustainable animal agriculture. There is never a one-size-fits-all when it comes to food, but having informed discussions about dietary choices can lead to more holistic and environmentally friendly practices.

Regenerative agriculture is a farming method designed to restore soil health, increase biodiversity, and enhance ecosystem resilience while producing nutrient-dense food. It is a farming practice that is quite transformational and at direct odds with conventional farming. While conventional farming tends to focus on monocultures, synthetic fertilizers, and pesticides, regenerative agriculture focuses on establishing soil health, enhancing biodiversity, and improving ecosystem functions, all while providing humane treatment to livestock. This is similar to the concept of the "circle of life," but proper animal farming restores the ecosystems rather than draws life out of them.

Here, every constituent part of the ecosystem is quite important—plants, animals, soil, and water coexist in the cycle. For instance, if animals feed on grasslands, they fertilize it with their excreta, activate plant growth, and propagate high diversity flora and fauna. In such holistic approaches, land nourishment is accompanied by enhanced resilience for the entire ecosystem.

One reason that regenerative agriculture is so exciting is the potential that it holds for carbon sequestration. Well-managed grazing lands can capture large amounts of carbon dioxide from the atmosphere, where it resides as CO_2 gas, and store it in the soil and live plants. Regenerative practices could mean a lower carbon footprint for foods produced by such methods compared with conventional farming.

For example, grass-fed beef raised on regenerative farms sequesters more carbon than is emitted throughout its life cycle, whereas conventionally raised beef frequently results in net carbon loss. Studies suggest that regenerative farming can sequester up to 100% of annual CO_2

emissions if implemented globally.[7] Meanwhile, conventional farming often relies on intensive tillage, monocropping, and heavy use of synthetic fertilizers and pesticides. These practices can lead to soil degradation to the point of sterile soil and increased greenhouse gas emissions. Conventional farming uses chemicals such as Glyphosate to eradicate weeds, genetically modified seeds that can grow in Glyphosate-treated areas, pesticides to eradicate insects, mammals, and "pests" that would otherwise damage crops, and fertilizers to promote growth.

Studies have found ALL these man-made chemicals (including plastics) in the human body. Glyphosate has been determined to be a "probable carcinogen to the human body" by The International Agency for Research on Cancer (IARC) in 2015; however, this is not considered Scientifically proven at this point. Conventional farming is also a significant contributor to global emissions, with around 13.7 billion tons of CO2 equivalent released annually.[8] This makes the difference between this innovative farming technique and conventional farming day and night, and the

---

[7]Moyer, J., Smith, A., Rui, Y., Hayden, J. (2020). Regenerative agriculture and the soil carbon solution [white paper]. (https://rodaleinstitute.org/wp-content/uploads/Rodale-Soil-Carbon-White-Paper_v11-compressed.pdf)
[8]Bianca Nogrady. (2024). How farming could become the ultimate climate-change tool. *Nature*. https://doi.org/10.1038/d41586-024-02036-x

environmental benefit of regenerative practices is enormous; therefore, it is an excellent reason for consumers to support those methods. The problem isn't consuming animals; it's about how we have chosen to produce animals for consumption. Although humanely raised animals that are grass-fed produce less meat, they are healthier for you and the environment.

In the case of dairy farming, with regenerative farming, cows graze on different pastures. This would ultimately ensure that they have a diverse diet that closely mirrors their natural eating behavior and could translate to healthier digestion and fewer incidents of illness. On regenerative farms, cows roam freely across pastures, their days spent grazing on diverse grasses, nursing their calves, and enjoying the sunlight—an existence far removed from the cramped, mechanized conditions of factory farming. Therefore, the cows are in better health because of all this and tend to produce higher-quality meats and milk.

Ruminants, such as cattle and sheep, are also critical components in maintaining grassland ecosystems. These animals are "Nature's lawnmowers and fertilizers." Being ruminants, they encourage growth control of plants by preventing a lush growth that could potentially fuel huge-scale fires and instead encourage rich growth of nutrient-contained grasses. Their grazing stimulates a range of plant life that supports all forms of wildlife. Their manure acts as a natural fertilizer, which will then enrich the soil, allowing it to retain more water. Regenerative farming does not contribute to desertification but contributes more to biodiversity and, thus, a well-balanced ecosystem of plant and animal life. Knowing and practicing regenerative agriculture becomes a way for farmers to utilize the inherent nature of ruminants in restoring or rejuvenating land in addition to supporting a healthier planet.

For our ancestors, animals were not just food but partners in survival. Their grazing patterns shaped the land, fertilized the soil, and supported plant life—an ancient symbiosis we can replicate today through regenerative agriculture. Regenerative agriculture is centered around sustainable farming practices that restore ecosystems, being different from traditional farming methods often known to degrade soil health and biodiversity.

In a regenerative approach, livestock becomes integral parts of the landscape beyond merely serving as food sources. Their grazing over the pastures fertilizes the soil through their waste, encourages and develops plant growth, and enhances carbon sequestration. This cycle is like how our ancestors used to live, hunting and gathering wild game for food and foraging on other sustenance sources.

If we follow our forefather's footsteps, we will find it in compliance with the carnivore diet, which upholds nutrient-rich animal products that our bodies have been designed to use. While most modern diets aim to require some doses of carbohydrates and processed foods, the carnivore diet may deliver some of the most fundamental nutrients in a form closest to being used by the body, which may be more beneficial to health.

In 2004, restaurateur Fergus Henderson published two seminal books in the United Kingdom on the subject: 'The Whole Beast: Nose to Tail Eating' and 'Nose to Tail Eating: A Kind of British Cooking.' By no means did Henderson coin the term nose-to-tail eating, but he brought it more into the mainstream of British cuisine and generated a movement toward a more sustainable, economical, and nutritious way of eating animals.

The crux behind Henderson's books was to make it easier for the ordinary consumer to eat generally discarded animal parts like offal, bones, skin, pig's head, pig's trotters, beef heart, tripe, and a variety of other innards. These books take the values of the paleo diet to a new stage and truly acknowledge our ancestors' ways and the ecological, economic, and personal benefits that we might reap from eating as they did. Today, foodies around the world devour delicacies prepared from unknown parts of an animal, but indigenous cultures never really stopped eating them as they progressed into modern times.

Celebrated foodies like the late great Anthony Bourdain helped bring this way of eating into the limelight by showing many cultural food traditions on television shows.

In other words, "nose-to-tail" eating defines the necessity of consuming the whole animal in the name of ethical meat consumption. Not only does this act reduce waste, but it also increases the sense of appreciation regarding what was used for food. Organ meats and less common cuts enable you to be principle-driven whilst adding to nutrition and flavor.

Organ meats, such as the liver, heart, or kidneys, are nutrient-rich and great sources of essential vitamins and minerals less abundant in meat, such as heme iron, vitamins A and B12, and CoQ10. Tips for incorporating these cuts include beginning with recipes that blend them into familiar dishes. You can incorporate liver pâté into spreads or add a heart to stews. This way, you promote a more sustainable use of meat by embracing the whole animal, allowing you to honor the life given and ensuring that nothing goes to waste.

But if we look at the real environmental costs behind our food choices, we must not look away from mono-crop agriculture. There seems to be a common narrative that veganism is the most environmentally friendly choice, but the truth might be another tale altogether.

Mono-crop farming tends to cause soil depletion, loss of biodiversity, and increased pesticide use, all having greater impacts on surrounding ecosystems. For instance, a single almond requires over a gallon of water to produce, making almond farming a significant contributor to water shortages in arid regions like California. Comparing the hidden cost, we can see how the environmental cost of foods like soy and almonds can sometimes be equal to that of grass-fed animals. For example, almonds require large amounts of water, are not very beneficial for the land, and often have great costs associated with it.

This type of knowledge for diet decisions encourages a more holistic approach to sustainability. There is a lot more to food than grabbing the best-looking bunch in the grocery store for healthy foods. A balanced approach involves the means of production, distribution, and environmental impact.

Thus, by choosing locally, sustainably sourced food, whether plant-based or animal-derived—we are making informed decisions that may support personal health and the planet's health. It is a matter of finding a balanced diet that supports the ecosystem and conserves natural resources responsibly. The path to sustainability isn't about choosing sides—it's about understanding the broader impact of our food systems and striving for practices that heal the planet.

This means being a "conscious carnivore," conscious not only of the treatment of the animal but also aware of how the meat is processed. Celebrity chef and world food traveler Anthony Bourdain was known for eating meat from head to tail, including organ meats, veal, and fish cheeks. He also enjoyed hotpot, pho, and sushi. A simple place to begin this journey is by learning to read a label successfully. Look for certifications from humane treatment and sustainable practices, such as "grass-fed," "pasture-raised," "certified humane, "American Grassfed Association," or "Certified Animal Welfare Approved." When shopping at your local farmers' markets or visiting farms, ask questions to learn more about the animal's life. Ask how the animals are fed and raised and whether any antibiotics or hormones are used. Find more information online at websites like EatWild.com or LocalHarvest.org.

Direct contact with producers encourages openness and trust. Third, there are local directories of farms, community-supported agriculture (CSA) programs, and Meat Shares, where consumers can search for contact with sustainable meat producers to make the process of access easier and thus ethically possible. Some examples of popular meat shares are Roxbury Farm, Garden of Eve, Devon Point Farm, North Mountain Pastures, and Bostrom Farm. Examples of regenerative agriculture include Butcher Block, White Oak Pastures, Flourish and Roam Farms, PatureBird, and others found here:

https://www.regenerativefarmersofamerica.com/regener ative-meats Coming to terms with food choices can be one of the most profound challenges in transitioning to ethical meat consumption. Many former vegetarians and vegans share their perspectives on ethical meat consumption; what becomes particularly evident is a shift in understanding and values.

They made several points that such a choice was based on a desire for health, ecological sustainability, and commitment to humane practice. In this light, people may come to understand their food choices and determine whether they have at their very core, a place of peace and direction in their lives. These stories serve as the embodiment of how a compassionate approach to eating can be approached with an appreciation for animals as well as concern for the earth.

The "Carnivore Carbon Footprint Challenge" offers an opportunity for consumers to equip themselves to measure and consequently minimize their personal carbon footprint when they are meat-eaters. It aims to make you introspective, take stock of the origin of their cuts of meat, and point out exactly where improvements can be made.

You can start on this challenge yourself by using carbon footprint calculators and guides for life cycles for different meats. These practices, combined with minimizing food waste by getting creative with leftovers and using fewer common cuts of meat, will push you to assist in reducing environmental impacts.

Supporting local and sustainable farming significantly impacts food systems; purchasing from farmers committed to regenerative practices keeps food systems strong. This way, you can still enjoy meat, reap the health benefits associated with a carnivore diet, and contribute positively to the environment—while doing so in line with your values.

Lastly, a carnivore diet related to the regenerative farming movement would also be a smart choice in that people can, therefore, enjoy healthy, high-quality animal foods and, at the same time, play their part in restoring ecosystems. This integrated approach pays homage to our ancestral eating patterns and sends a message that ensures a safe future on our planet, making it a well-thought-out case for those on the lookout for both personal health and ecological harmony. Choosing ethically raised, sustainably sourced meat isn't just about dinner—it's about casting your vote for a future where humans and the planet thrive together. Are you ready to take charge toward a healthier, more harmonious world?

Chapter 12: Science or Science Fiction? The Cutting Edge of Carnivore Research

Imagine a world in which doctors prescribe steak instead of statins and where nutritionists recommend ribeye over rice. It sounds like science fiction, right? Welcome to the cutting edge of carnivore research, where today's radical notions might just become tomorrow's new normal.

My personal experience when being diagnosed with pre-diabetes was a prescription for Metformin and also an SSRI [which is the current medical guideline in the United States]. I was not offered another option. I needed to request information about other non-medication options, such as diet and exercise. I was told that those were options but warned that if my tests did not improve, I would need to reconsider the lifelong medication route. I chose the dietary change, and to this day, I am no longer considered diabetic.

To understand meat-based diets, it appears that researchers are busying themselves to conduct studies that enlighten us on the potential benefits and risks associated with this diet. Some recent observational studies[9] found diets high in red and processed meat to be positively associated with health risks like cardiovascular disease and colorectal cancer; however, the other[10] says protein-rich diets have benefits for maintaining muscle mass among older adults.

It is the bipolar nature of people's opinions and research findings that create hesitation among people to try any new diet that they are not familiar with. Things just become more complex when it comes to clinical trials. Although some short-term studies come in with a glamorized stance on plant-based diets related to weight loss and better metabolic profiles, these usually have caveats attached: they are often focused on immediate effects rather than long-term health outcomes. In this material landscape of evidence, I hope to sift through to find the gems that shine a light on how meat-based diets affect human health for the better.

As this diet becomes more popular, quite a few researchers have taken an interest in studying its implications. Presently, ongoing studies are researching

---

[9] Frank Qian, Matthew C. Riddle, Judith Wylie-Rosett, Frank B. Hu; Red and Processed Meats and Health Risks: How Strong Is the Evidence?. Diabetes Care 1 February 2020; 43 (2): 265–271. https://doi.org/10.2337/dci19-0063
[10] Putra C, Konow N, Gage M, York CG, Mangano KM. Protein Source and Muscle Health in Older Adults: A Literature Review. Nutrients. 2021; 13(3):743. https://doi.org/10.3390/nu13030743

the impact on different health parameters, including inflammatory markers, gut microbiota, and mental conditions. Studies, such as 'Can a carnivore diet provide all essential nutrients?'[11] are conducted to discuss the diet's potential benefits and health risks.

A lot of people share anecdotal evidence, and various famous individuals have attested to doing quite well on strict carnivorous diets, but this doesn't replace scientific investigation. Ongoing research is important to be designed to rigorously assess long-term effects and how this diet works. The excitement around this area of research does bet an evolution in nutrition science: one that grows more responsive to real-world dietary practices and acknowledges the thousands of people who swear by a carnivore diet.

However, the dynamics of a study involving a carnivore diet [and any nutrition-based study] pose unique methodological challenges that are akin to navigating a scientific obstacle course. Participant recruitment is one of the major hurdles since strict adherents to a carnivore diet are small, self-selected groups, making representative samples hard to gather.

---

[11] O'Hearn A. Can a carnivore diet provide all essential nutrients? Curr Opin Endocrinol Diabetes Obes. 2020 Oct;27(5):312-316. doi: 10.1097/MED.0000000000000576. PMID: 32833688.

Long-term diet studies are also not easy logistically. It takes quite a lot of time and input to follow up for long periods, and participants are likely to go off their assigned diets, thus complicating the analysis of data. Again, in diet studies, there is the confounding variable factor of genetics and lifestyle, which at times would mask the diet's effect on its own.

Though the potential gain of the findings is promising in studying this carnivore diet, scientists must hold their breath while trying to navigate these unknown waters. As they learn to better manage the boundaries in the science of nutrition, there may eventually be a revelation of whether such a polarizing approach to diet, i.e., carnivore diet, is a nutritional boon or a hidden pitfall. Until that time comes, this is a potential method that can be used to better understand the effect of a carnivore diet in a scientific manner.

Self-experimentation in Meat-based Diets

Case studies and N=1 experiments—where individuals keep a record of their health outcomes—generate a rich source of insights into meat-based diets. Many practitioners of the carnivore diet have documented personal journeys, transforming energy levels, body composition, and overall well-being. Although self-reports or anecdotal experiences often reveal patterns that are consistent in individuals, these observations still warrant scientific investigation. For instance, there was one fellow, Harris, with autoimmune problems who went on an impressive decline in symptoms while following a complete carnivorous diet. Maintaining very precise self-observations, changes in inflammation markers, mood, and even exercise performance were tracked to later be analyzed. Such anecdotes show how self-experimentation might eventually give us momentum in terms of the knowledge to be gained regarding diet-induced effects, even though personal accounts are not to be considered as law or fact.

In the process of finding a balanced view, there is a need to debunk common myths surrounding health issues related to the carnivore diet. Let's look at some of the most common myths and provide evidence-based refutations.

Myth-busting Served with Science

1. **Cardiovascular Health:** Critics often cite the link between saturated fat and heart disease. However, recent meta-analyses challenge this connection, suggesting no significant relationship when saturated fats are consumed within whole-food-based diets. For example, a 2020 meta-analysis in *The American Journal of Clinical Nutrition* found no conclusive evidence tying dietary saturated fat to

increased cardiovascular risk. New research[12] suggests that the relationship between saturated fats and heart health may not be as cut-and-dried as previously believed, going as far as to indicate that no increased risk of cardiovascular disease was observed when saturated fats are part of a whole-food diet. One must question whether the public has been steered away from natural animal products and driven towards more profitable, industrialized, highly processed food solutions through marketing, lobbying, and regulation.

2. **Cancer Risk:** While processed meats are classified as carcinogenic by the WHO, unprocessed animal products show a different profile. Diets minimizing carbohydrates may reduce insulin and IGF-1 levels, potentially lowering cancer risk. A study published in *Cell Metabolism* highlights how reduced carbohydrate intake influences these pathways. Proponents argue that the absence of carbohydrates may naturally reduce levels of insulin, the hormone implicated in some types of cancer. Therefore, more studies need to determine such associations to strengthen the literature review on this particular topic.

---

[12] Malhotra A, Redberg RF, Meier PSaturated fat does not clog the arteries: coronary heart disease is a chronic inflammatory condition, the risk of which can be effectively reduced from healthy lifestyle interventions British Journal of Sports Medicine 2017;51:1111-1112.

3. **Micronutrient Deficiency:** The biggest argument on the part of critics is that people are easily prone to vitamin and mineral deficiencies following a carnivore diet. Meanwhile, followers of this diet hold the view that one could achieve nutrient density by including a diversified range of animal products. For example, organ meats are highly nutrient-dense and could counterbalance such deficiencies with vitamins like B12, and A and essential minerals such as zinc and selenium. For example, 100g of beef liver offers more vitamin A than most plant-based foods.

4. **Longevity:** Sure, some studies[13] are saying that those who follow a plant-based diet live longer, but mounting evidence simply states that well-formulated carnivore diets are just as effective and that following a plant-based diet does not necessarily affect the mortality rate. Recently, researchers have emphasized quality of life and metabolic health as just as important to longevity as diet.

This all might seem a bit daunting, but understanding how a carnivore diet might improve health involves

---

[13] Norman K, Klaus S. Veganism, aging and longevity: new insight into old concepts. Curr Opin Clin Nutr Metab Care. 2020 Mar;23(2):145-150. doi: 10.1097/MCO.0000000000000625. PMID: 31895244.

exploring several biological mechanisms. Here's a simplified look at a few:

1. **Reduced Inflammation:** A low-carb diet high in healthy fats may decrease pro-inflammatory markers in the body. This could be attributed to removing specific antigens from plant foods, potentially benefiting people with inflammatory conditions.

2. **Increased Satiety and Insulin Sensitivity:** High-protein diets make you feel fuller for a long time, regulating blood sugar levels. Carnivore removes the up and down spikes associated with high-carb, high-sugar intake diets. Reducing carbohydrate intake might also increase your insulin sensitivity—the factor by which you can prevent type 2 diabetes.

3. **Gut Health:** Some proponents of the carnivore diet claim it can support gut health without relying on fiber. A diet rich in proteins and fats can exhibit prebiotic effects, feeding beneficial gut bacteria and potentially increasing beneficial cell growth and health in the intestines. Another benefit of this elimination diet is the removal of processed food ingredients related to "leaky gut" syndromes.

Leaky gut syndrome

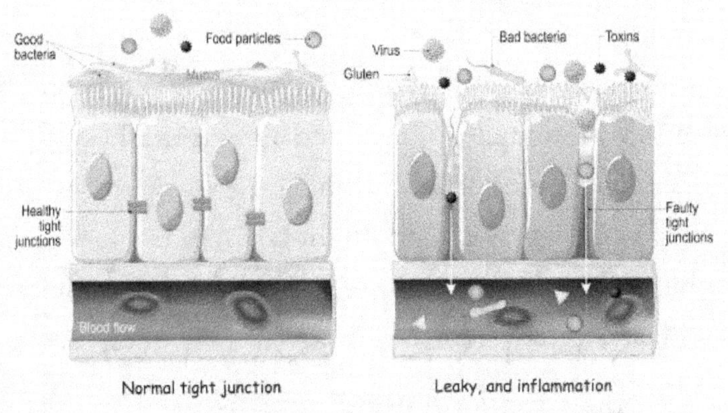

As the carnivore diet remains a health question, research must continue, self-experimentation should thrive, and biological mechanisms must be understood. By relating anecdotal evidence with scientific inquiry, we can continue to untangle the pieces of meat-based diets and make them more accessible to the general public.

With the increased popularity of this diet, newer research areas with lots of promise are gaining traction. Perhaps the most exciting one is **Nutrigenomics**, the study of how genetic variations between individuals interact to modify their responses to nutrients. Nutrigenomics attempts to provide individually tailored dietary guidance for people based on their genetic makeup. For dieters following a carnivorous diet, knowing how genes impact metabolism, nutrient absorption, and health in general could open new avenues toward individualized approaches.

Emerging research on this topic can explain reasons why some genetic polymorphisms might benefit from the utilization of animal proteins and fats in the body. This way, we can determine who would be good candidates for a carnivorous diet and who might not stand it. It will also emphasize the personal nature of nutrition and how each individual is different.

The other frontier research topic is the discovery of **Ancestral Microbiomes**. That means learning about the gut bacteria of our ancestors and how the modern diet interacts with these ecosystems. It may bring findings about how much a meat-based diet affects human evolution and health; in other words, evidence of a balance of microbes that thrived on high-meat diets and how contemporary diets, including plant-heavy approaches, alter gut health.

Researchers aim to compare microbiomes to understand the benefits of a meat-centric diet for a healthy gut, focusing on contemporary carnivore dieters versus traditional hunter-gatherer societies. Although promising, it is also important to critically evaluate the limitations of a carnivore diet. To this end, here are key criticisms, limitations, and areas that require further study:

1. **Very Few Long-term Studies:** Most of the carnivore diet studies are observational or anecdotal, and very few long-term, prospective clinical studies report on the safety and efficacy of this diet. Only rigorous studies allow us to generalize results, which are currently lacking in the carnivore diet.

2. **Self-selection Bias:** The people reporting positive outcomes with the carnivore diet are very self-motivated and have been influenced to try out this diet, which skews results. Creating a more accurate data set is important and, therefore, requires the use of larger study groups, which will be more representative.

3. **Nutrient Variability:** Some argue that the nutrient content of animal products is extremely high, but animal sources vary greatly in nutrient profiles, and individual diets also depend on specific eating habits.

4. **Potential Health Risks:** While there are researchers who have pointed out the beneficial effects of consuming meat, there are also those who are conducting studies into risks in the long-term on kidney health and bone density because of excessive intake of meat.

5. **Individual Variation in Reactions:** People react differently to a diet of only meat. All these factors come under genetics, the constitution of the microbiome, and past health issues that play a role in individual results,

which brought about the conclusion that there cannot be an all-around fit for everybody in terms of diet.

6. **Confounding Factors:** Many studies do not adequately control for confounding factors, such as genetics, lifestyle, and other dietary habits, making it difficult to isolate the effects of the carnivore diet. Robust methodologies are needed to account for these variables and get accurate findings.

7. **Conflicts of Interest:** Big Food and Big Pharma are among the largest advertisers and supporters of media, lobbyists, medical education, and politicians. These companies are judged by their bottom lines financially. It is against their best interest to promote natural foods and a healthier population that does not lean on highly processed foods and lifelong medications. Many health studies are paid for by this industry. Guess which way the outcomes of these studies incline. Try this yourself by asking this question to ChatGPT:

Did cigarette scientists go to work for the big food industry?

ChatGPT said:

ChatGPT

Yes, there is evidence that scientists and marketing experts who worked for the tobacco industry transitioned to roles within the food industry. This shift occurred largely during the latter half of the 20th century, particularly as the tobacco industry faced increasing regulation and public scrutiny.

Key Points:

1. Tobacco Tactics Adapted for Food:

o The tobacco industry mastered strategies to downplay health risks and promote addictive products. Some of these tactics, like manipulating public perception and lobbying against regulation, were later employed by the food industry to market processed foods, sugary products, and snacks.

o Scientists and executives who specialized in manipulating flavor profiles and addictive properties of tobacco products used similar techniques to develop hyper-palatable, highly processed foods designed to maximize consumption.

2. Shared Marketing and Lobbying Techniques:

o Former tobacco marketers and lobbyists applied their skills in shaping public opinion, creating doubt about scientific evidence, and influencing policy to protect the food industry's interests.

o The food industry has been accused of funding research to minimize the perceived harm of sugar, salt, and fat—similar to how tobacco companies funded studies that downplayed smoking risks.

3. Examples:

- o In the 1980s and 1990s, major food companies like Kraft, General Foods, and Philip Morris were linked. Philip Morris owned Kraft and General Foods, and their marketing expertise from tobacco influenced food marketing strategies.

- o The creation of "bliss point" foods, which combine sugar, salt, and fat to trigger dopamine responses in the brain, is one example of how these methods were applied.

Consequences:

- These practices have been linked to the rise of chronic health issues such as obesity, diabetes, and heart disease.

- Some researchers and health advocates argue that the food industry's behavior parallels the tobacco industry's history of prioritizing profits over public health.

This history highlights the importance of scrutinizing how industries influence public health and consumer behavior.

I said: Hmmmm, that is interesting.

As much as we aim to clear out misunderstandings, it is important to acknowledge criticism of this nature as it enables readers to have a well-rounded view of the carnivore diet and stay well-informed with future emerging studies. Only once you have understood all sides of the argument can you fully accept this diet without any reservations.

However, for researchers interested in future research into the carnivore diet, these could be among potential areas to look into:

1. **Longitudinal Studies:** Properly designed long studies with long-term monitoring of health outcomes among a varied group of individuals following the carnivore diet.

2. **Nutritional Analysis:** Determining if the diet is adequate in its supply of nutrients, what deficiencies are likely to arise, and how these can be prevented or minimized.

3. **Mechanisms of Action:** Examining what biological mechanisms of the carnivore diet may or may not affect the health condition of the individual, especially concerning inflammation, metabolism, and gut integrity.

4. **Expanding Demographics**: Carry out studies involving more diverse participant demographics to get a clearer view of how the diet performs on other demographics than the usual participants.

5. **Quality of Life Studies:** Measure better overall well-being as well as quality of life in research to use as a better all-around picture of the diet's effect.

By addressing some criticisms and focusing on these areas, future research can work to provide a more well-rounded understanding of the carnivore diet and its possible health effects. Now that we have a better understanding of this topic and its research standing, you can take this quiz to test your knowledge. To solidify key concepts from this chapter, here is the 'Are You a Carnivore Science Whiz?' quiz. Read each question and answer by selecting from the given options. In the end, check the answer key to see how well you understood the concept of this chapter.

1. What is nutrigenomics?

A. The study of how diet affects gut microbiota

B. How genetic factors influence nutritional requirements to be determined

C. Analysis of diets past

2. Among the latest research findings, which of the following is a benefit associated with an animal-product-containing diet?

A. Higher sugar cravings

B. Enhanced insulin sensitivity

C. Higher fatigue

3. Why is self-experimentation relevant to carnivore diet studies?

A. It established a scientific standard

B. It provides anecdotal evidence of responses from individuals

C. It trumps the need for clinical trials

4. Which of the following is a criticism of the diet?

A) It has extensive long-term studies behind it

B) It may produce nutrient deficiencies

C) That is applauded by nutrition experts with one voice

5. 5. How would ancestral microbiome research help us understand the carnivore diet?

A) As a comparison between modern diets and those of the earliest humans

B) By proving that plant-based diets are superior

C) By dismissing the importance of gut health

Answer Key: 1. B 2. B 3. B 4. B 5. A

In fully exploring these ideas, readers can enrich their knowledge of the current and continually changing state of science regarding carnivore diet research and be updated with new research and any emerging findings.

Chapter 13: Thriving in a Carb-crazed World: Your Social Survival Guide

Imagine you are at an entertaining party, heavy with the noise of chatter, laughter, and the delicious aroma coming from a variety of food options. You look at the buffet table, where you are met with an endless ocean of carbohydrate-rich choices. You see a mountain of pasta salad, towering slices of cake, and a variety of desserts that can easily pull even the strongest of wills. And as others sit down to a sugary feast, you huddle over your plate of cold cuts like a life raft in a turbulent sea.

Fear not, brave meat-eater, for I am here to guide you through the waters and help you become a master of social survival. With this final guide, you will become a pro in cutting through a sea of carbohydrates easily and confidently with this **Carnivore Comeback 101.**

It is, therefore, important that when curious onlookers, such as friends and family or even acquaintances, raise an eyebrow about your dietary choices, you are armed with thoughtfully worded and tactful responses. Imagine this scenario: someone leans over the table, glances at your plate, and says, "Why don't you just eat some salad?" Instead of feeling cornered or defensive, you could respond graciously and assuredly. A good reply would be, "Really appreciate the offer!

Actually, I found that my body thrives with a carnivore diet; it just works wonders regarding energy levels and overall health. But the food options are great, and I am glad you are enjoying it." I usually reply that I am doing my "Carnivore Experiment" and want to stay true to the process.

This approach expresses your choice of food but also lets the conversation turn pleasant instead of turning into a debate. It will also encourage them to ask you questions without making you feel guilty about making your food choices.

Now, suppose the discussion leads to the topic of concerns over the loss of quality nutrients. In that case, you can simply respond by saying this: "Many people don't realize that nutrient density in animal products is much higher and can actually fulfill most of the requirements one has." It lightens the conversation about nutrients and lets others know that you are indeed informed and educated about your choices in terms of diet and nutrition.

Food is not just a medium of nourishment; it holds deep emotional significance and cultural context. Diet debate often becomes an identity issue, a historical matter, and a matter of emotional connection with people. The conversations concerning diet can often become emotionally charged and can turn into tense discussions.

To avoid that and to understand the emotional landscape, you may say, "I see that my diet choice raises some concerns for you. Curiosity is just another way of showing you care. If you have any questions, I am happy to answer them for you." This can diffuse potential tension and encourage a respectful dialogue by acknowledging their feelings.

You can also share your personal journey and what inspires you to live this way, which may make other people understand and connect better. Instead of discouraging them from inquiring about your diet, invite them into your story as you explain how you began to appreciate the benefits brought about by a carnivorous diet through personal experience and research. You can also mention the health improvements you experienced after following this new diet.

By letting them know that your choices are not a judgment of their eating habits, you can find out the commonality between your preferences and interests beyond the confines of the plate. This strengthens relationships between friends and helps individuals feel at home despite their diets. We talked a bit about parties and social gatherings, but Dining Out as a carnivore is often like a strategic operation— an adventure in culinary exploration.

To help make that easy for yourself, just pick places that specialize in meat dishes. Steakhouses and BBQ joints are the best, with plenty of things to order from the menu that align with your diet preference. Alternatively, consider American diners or Asian cuisines, among others, who have different menus with grilled meats. In these kinds of restaurants, you can freely get creative about your ordering. For example, you may order a ribeye at a steakhouse served with extra meat and nothing else. You will realize that so many restaurants are quite open-minded about special orders.

In diners or burger joints, you can order a beef burger without the buns or just order the beef patties on their own. Personally, I order 2 beef patties, cheese, and bacon on each, no bun. Are you craving sushi and dining at a sushi place? Order sashimi instead of the rolls to avoid the rice. These minor changes will ensure that you stay on your carnivore diet path and are able to navigate social environments and restaurants comfortably and confidently.

Prepping for social events can be fun and daunting at the same time, but a little advanced planning will make all the difference in your experience at social gatherings. One great tip is to find out ahead of time what food will be served. If you find that options are limited or heavily rely on carbs, prepare a tasty meal ahead of time to avoid undesirable non-carnivore foods. One of the best approaches to ensure that you get something to eat at whatever event is always to come prepared with a cooler in hand.

Picture this: a small cooler filled with delectable, sliced meats, cheeses, or homemade treats, all aligned according to your personal dietary decisions. Having your own snacks will ensure you won't ever starve, but it also opens the possibility of sharing your tasty snacks with others to create curiosity and talk about your diet journey.

If you are offered food that doesn't align with your diet, you can decline it politely when someone offers you choices that do not have anything to do with what you eat. Here, for example, a polite way of saying this could be, "Thanks so much for thinking of me, but I need to keep my diet. Thanks so much for your understanding!"

For all the travel enthusiasts, a carnivore diet is quite a rewarding adventure as you get to try new cuisines and flavors. Research the local food options before you go traveling to discover more options in other cultures. Grilled meat is a staple in many places, and it should be easily incorporated into your dietary needs. Besides that, a few words of the local lingo can take you far in ordering well while out of the country. Learn a few key phrases related to meat dishes in the local language. This, of course, not only makes the meals taste better but also ties you closer to the culture.

Use apps such as Yelp or TripAdvisor to find restaurants and markets that are friendly to carnivores so you will be able to enjoy great meals and not stray from your food choices. Do not shy away from visiting local butcheries and farms for fresh, healthy meat products. Most of these businesses have specialties that cater specifically to your dietary needs; therefore, you can consider visiting such places for even more meaningful travel experiences.

Getting up close and personal with butchers or the farmer himself may be quite a jackpot when it comes to discovering new foods, even for the most seasoned epicurean. Armed with these insights and strategies, you're prepared to survive the next party and become a confident carnivore in a world filled with many different diets.

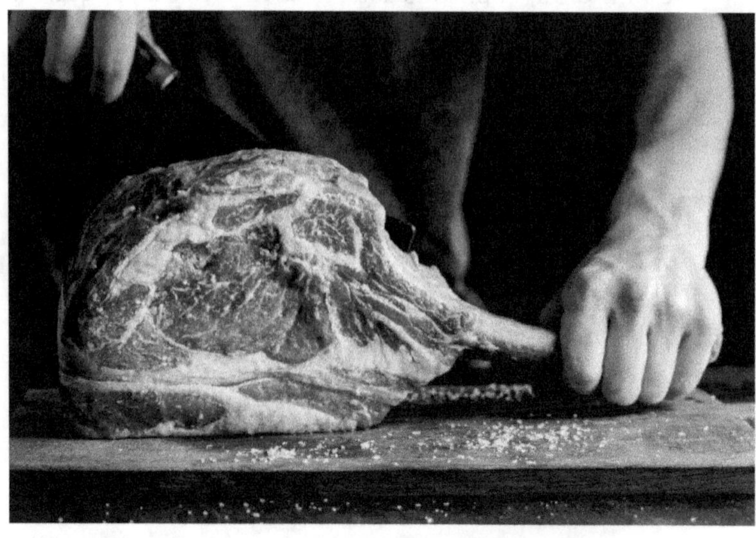

Maintaining an exclusive meat diet in challenging environments, including college dorms, military service, or cohabitation with non-carnivorous family members, requires creativity and prior planning. For a student in a college, the available kitchen space may be minimal, but having a mini fridge and a microwave can be useful in storing and preparing relatively simple meat dishes. Convenient foods to consume are quite easily available, including cooked sausages or other canned meats, and one may stock these for quick preparation. If you are in the military, prepping in advance and storing food in vacuum bags will ensure that the food is fresh when you arrive at your destination.

You might be living with family members who have different eating habits. The way you solve this is through open communication about what you want to eat. You can engage your family members to help you in planning meals by suggesting foods that are versatile and easy to adjust for the case, or you can prepare your own carnivorous food and prepare their different diets for the day.

With an active attitude and these effective tips, you can rock at any social interaction while remaining true to your dietary needs. Having a supportive community and many like-minded people increases camaraderie and potential motivation. To find or join local meetups, give platforms like Meetup.com or Facebook groups on a carnivore diet a try. These sites host multiple events like casual get-togethers and potlucks where one can mingle with like-minded folks.

If there isn't one, then start your own. Organizing monthly meetups in a park near your home or cooking classes based on carnivore recipes might be quite amusing. Online, you can find fine resources for sharing recipes, tips, and success stories across social media platforms, such as Instagram and Reddit, and specialized forums that allow you to engage with a larger community and learn from others' experiences.

Advocating for the carnivore diet is something of an art. How you tell your story without coming off as preachy, divisive, or exclusionary, yet still introducing people to your way of life, can be a fine line to walk. Be empathetic and respectful in your approach during the conversation. When someone asks you about your diet, do not say that it is the best diet, but instead, speak of your experience and the positive changes you've seen because of it. You could say this: "I have found that a carnivore diet really works for me because…"

Hear what they have to say and be considerate of their diets because everyone needs and likes something different. You can make others curious about the carnivore diet but do not alarm others by being open-minded and judgment-free when discussing it. In that manner, you help create a climate that welcomes question and exploration rather than resistance. Own these choices, converse productively with others, and remember that every social gathering is an opportunity to share your dietary preferences and your personal journey and experiences. With encouragement to be more empathetic, understanding, and interested in learning about what's happening, difficulties imposed by social dining would soon be overcome with deeper connections built with others around. So, step boldly into that room filled with people and take up the delectable task of being a carnivore in the sea of carbs.

Let's take the example of Amanda, who has now become a pro at navigating social situations. According to Amanda, for the past four years, her family has alternated between being ketogenic and not. She has five children with her spouse, and they have their own difficulties. Her 12-year-old son has autism, in addition to having weak muscle tone, excessive thirst, and inexplicable weight loss since adolescence. Amanda believed she needed to begin healing herself and her family after watching videos about the carnivore diet.

Her autistic youngster consumed a lot of almond milk and carbohydrates. Her middle daughter was constantly requesting rice or spaghetti since she was a carbohydrate addict. Her girls all possessed a "very bad sweet tooth."

"It kind of freaked me out because my son had all the symptoms of a type 1 diabetic," Amanda says after seeing a video about the disease. When she brought her son to the doctor for a checkup, the physician declared him to be in good health; however, Amanda didn't believe it.

About three weeks into their carnivore month, Amanda strayed from her usual diet and placed an order for pizza one evening. After eating some, her son had a "massive meltdown" the following day. Calming him down took several days.

In another instance, Amanda and her family enjoyed some cake and cookies for dessert after dinner at a friend's house. The children experienced severe stomachaches that night, and by morning, they were feeling extremely nauseous. It was then that Amanda discovered that her family was unable to tolerate processed foods.

Amanda says that eating carnivore-style food is a way of life. She and her husband explained to family and friends that eating this way is important, especially for their son, who has special needs. Although they found this diet to be unconventional and judged Amanda for 'forcing' her kids to eat like this, she stuck with this diet.

It took her middle daughter time to adjust to no carbs, but she is now the biggest steak eater in the family. Now, the family consumes a lot of meat, eggs, and dairy, and Amanda uses cheese and heavy cream with eggs to provide fat for the kids, whereas raw milk yogurt serves as a snack. The veggies have gradually faded from the family's meals completely and been replaced by animal-based side dishes.

Conclusion: Your Meaty Destiny Awaits

Well, dear reader, we've finally reached the end of our meaty journey. But remember, this is merely the beginning of your carnivore adventure. Your destiny—a healthier, happier, meat-powered you—awaits! As we part ways, let's recap some of the key takeaways that will guide you as your "Carnivore Commandments."

1. Know the reasons behind your dietary choice in order to make your commitment stronger. I like the phrase, "I'm eating for my health, not my pleasure."

2. Make plans for social situations in advance so that you will be able to have an enjoyable time and enjoy yourself within the confines of your diet. I have found this to be a conversation starter, which is usually well-received.

3. Find a community. Local or online carnivore groups may aid you in getting their support and inspiration. YouTube has a large community. I started with "SteakAndButterGal."

4. A Carnivore should be an advocate of the diet but respect the choices of others. Practice, not Preach. This one takes some skill. I get so enthusiastic about explaining the diet that I need to remind myself to position it in a way that is my healthy choice, which I am happy to tell you about without preaching to you to follow this lifestyle.

My hope is to give you some good points to consider in your own health journey.

5. There is no single formula; you simply need to explore and find what works best for your body and lifestyle. Every person is different, and what works for others may not work for you. This is particularly important! If you take away key concepts of eating in a more natural way, you will be in a much better position health-wise.

6. Measure the results from more dimensions than the scale, including overall healthy being and energy. Check for mental clarity, energy, stamina, medical tests, and more.

7. Stay Educated. Continue reading about new research and breakthroughs in meat-based nutrition to perfect your plan. There are many videos online that go over the pros and cons of carnivore, paleo, vegetarian, and vegan diets. I encourage you to review them all with an open mind and make decisions on your own. What is common between them all? That answer is a more natural diet!

8. Hone in on the game plan, develop strategies for setbacks, and resist the temptation of reverting back to unhealthy habits.

9. Most importantly, have realistic expectations and give the diet some time to work its magic. I saw changes in 2 weeks, a significant reduction in blood sugar levels in

90 days, and significant benefits (weight loss, body recomposition, reduced blood pressure, fewer skin issues) in 1 year.

As with any bespoke carnivore plan, remember that personalization is important, so be prepared to try new things that fit your needs. What works for someone else might not work for you, and again, it's okay to adapt the solution as the situation presents itself. Realistic expectations and goals in achieving well-being, not just losing weight, are important. Set up a specific "Carnivore Success Plan" tailored to one's own needs. Keep track of achievements regarding improving energy levels, mood, or improving health.

Nutrition is not a fixed topic; it's a never-ending series of improvements and updates. Stay current with what new research is coming out through reputable books, podcasts, or online courses on the topic of carnivore diets and meat-based nutrition. All these will help you decide better and adjust your eating habits as needed.

And as you go through the ebbs and flows of this journey, do not forget that plateaus or setbacks do not mean you failed. Indeed, they simply call for reassessing your goals and strategies and staying the course while reminding yourself of the many benefits of staying free from carbs and processed foods.

This diet might not be the norm now, but growing interest in the carnivore diet could open up "Meat-opia" in the future, where choices of how to eat meat are not only available but also respected. With some imagination, think about a future when restaurants have diversified menus centered around meat, grocery stores brimming with excellent meats, and healthcare systems embracing the benefits of meat-based nutrition.

As you progress on this path, let yourself become an evangelist for the lifestyle of the carnivore. Share all your successes, insights, and the life-changing benefits you have discovered. Personal testimony brings value that inspires others to explore different food choices and further down a path that sets conventionality aside.

Thank you for joining the meat revolution. It takes guts, quite literally, to question the status quo and take one's own health decisions into their hands. Every gathering, every meal out, and every conversation is an opportunity to share not just your plate but your journey. By embracing curiosity and empathy, you show the world that your choices are rooted in health and personal growth, not in judgment or exclusion. So, as you step into the carb-crazed world, know that your journey as a carnivore is about much more than food—it's about thriving authentically, fostering connection, and living your truth unapologetically.

References

1. O'Keefe, J. H., et al. "Dietary strategies for cardiovascular disease prevention: focus on dietary fats and cholesterol." The Lancet Diabetes & Endocrinology (2019).

2. Cordain, L., et al. "Origins and evolution of the Western diet: health implications for the 21st century." The American Journal of Clinical Nutrition (2005).

3. Milton, K. "A hypothesis to explain the role of meat-eating in human evolution." Evolutionary Anthropology (1999).

4. Sayers, K. "Human evolution and the ancestral human diet: Insights from hominid biology." Quarterly Review of Biology (2016).

5. Ungar, P. S. "Dental evidence for diet in early hominins." Philosophical Transactions of the Royal Society B: Biological Sciences (2012).

6. Bell, J. G., et al. "Meat-eating and human evolution." Nature (2009).

7. Hockett, B., Haws, J. "Carnivory in the carnivores: The role of meat-eating in human evolution." Evolutionary Anthropology (2014).

8. Aiello, L., Wheeler, P. "The Expensive Tissue Hypothesis: The brain and the digestive system in human and primate evolution." Current Anthropology (1995).

9. Milton, K. "Nutritional characteristics of wild primate foods: do the diets of our closest living relatives have lessons for us?" Nutrition (1999).

10. Wells, J. C. K. "The evolution of human fatness and susceptibility to obesity: An ethological approach." Biological Reviews (2006).

11. Wrangham, R. "Catching fire: how cooking made us human." Basic Books (2009).

12. Stefansson, V. "The Fat of the Land: The Inuit Diet." Harper & Row (1956).

13. Mann, G. V., et al. "Diet and cardiovascular risk in the Maasai." The American Journal of Epidemiology (1972).

14. Kuipers, R. S., et al. "Estimated macronutrient and fatty acid intake from an East African Paleolithic diet." The British Journal of Nutrition (2010).

15. Wrangham, R., Conklin-Brittain, N. "Cooking as a biological trait." Comparative Biochemistry and Physiology (2003).

16. Crawford, M. A., et al. "Fatty acid ratios in free-living and domestic animals: Implications for human diet and health." Proceedings of the Nutrition Society (2009).

17. Lieberman, D. E. "The Story of the Human Body: Evolution, Health, and Disease." Pantheon (2013).

18. Cordain, L., et al. "Plant-animal subsistence ratios and macronutrient energy estimations in worldwide hunter-gatherer diets." The American Journal of Clinical Nutrition (2000).

19. Malhotra A, Redberg RF, Meier P. Saturated fat does not clog the arteries: coronary heart disease is a chronic inflammatory condition, the risk of which can be effectively reduced from healthy lifestyle interventions, British Journal of Sports Medicine 2017;51:1111-1112.

20. Vesnina A, Prosekov A, Kozlova O, Atuchin V. Genes and Eating Preferences, Their Roles in Personalized Nutrition. Genes (Basel). 2020 Mar 27;11(4):357. doi: 10.3390/genes11040357. PMID: 32230794; PMCID: PMC7230842.

21. Zajac A, Poprzecki S, Maszczyk A, Czuba M, Michalczyk M, Zydek G. The Effects of a Ketogenic Diet on Exercise Metabolism and Physical Performance in Off-Road Cyclists. Nutrients. 2014; 6(7):2493-2508. https://doi.org/10.3390/nu6072493.

22. Dobersek U, Teel K, Altmeyer S, Adkins J, Wy G, Peak J. Meat, and mental health: A meta-analysis of meat consumption, depression, and anxiety. Crit Rev Food Sci Nutr. 2023;63(19):3556-3573. doi: 10.1080/10408398.2021.1974336. Epub 2021 Oct 6. PMID: 34612096.

23. Leroy F, Smith NW, Adesogan AT, Beal T, Iannotti L, Moughan PJ, Mann N. The role of meat in the human diet: evolutionary aspects and nutritional value. Anim Front. 2023 Apr 15;13(2):11-18. doi: 10.1093/af/vfac093. PMID: 37073319; PMCID: PMC10105836.

24. Firth J, Veronese N, Cotter J, Shivappa N, Hebert JR, Ee C, Smith L, Stubbs B, Jackson SE, Sarris J. What Is the Role of Dietary Inflammation in Severe Mental Illness? A Review of Observational and Experimental Findings. Front Psychiatry. 2019 May 15;10:350. doi: 10.3389/fpsyt.2019.00350. PMID: 31156486; PMCID: PMC6529779.

25. Moyer, J., Smith, A., Rui, Y., Hayden, J. (2020). Regenerative agriculture and the soil carbon solution

[white paper]. (https://rodaleinstitute.org/wp-content/uploads/Rodale-Soil-Carbon-White-Paper_v11-compressed.pdf)

26. Frank Qian, Matthew C. Riddle, Judith Wylie-Rosett, Frank B. Hu; Red and Processed Meats and Health Risks: How Strong Is the Evidence?. Diabetes Care 1 February 2020; 43 (2): 265–271. https://doi.org/10.2337/dci19-0063

27. Putra C, Konow N, Gage M, York CG, Mangano KM. Protein Source and Muscle Health in Older Adults: A Literature Review. Nutrients. 2021; 13(3):743. https://doi.org/10.3390/nu13030743

28. O'Hearn A. Can a carnivore diet provide all essential nutrients? Curr Opin Endocrinol Diabetes Obes. 2020 Oct;27(5):312-316. doi: 10.1097/MED.0000000000000576. PMID: 32833688.

29. Malhotra A, Redberg RF, Meier PSaturated fat does not clog the arteries: coronary heart disease is a chronic inflammatory condition, the risk of which can be effectively reduced from healthy lifestyle interventions. Journal of Sports Medicine 2017;51:1111-1112.

30. Norman K, Klaus S. Veganism, aging, and longevity: new insight into old concepts. Curr Opin Clin Nutr Metab Care. 2020 Mar;23(2):145-150. doi: 10.1097/MCO.0000000000000625. PMID: 31895244.

31. Roundtable discussion: American Health & Nutrition: A Second Opinion hosted by Senator Ron Johnson September 25, 2024 https://youtu.be/rxz6VK9xJpg

32. The Groundbreaking Cancer Expert: (New Research)
    "This Common Food Is Making Cancer Worse!" Dr
    Thomas Seyfried is a professor of biology, genetics, and
    biochemistry at Boston College. He has over 150 peer-
    reviewed publications and is also the author of books
    such as, 'Cancer as a Metabolic Disease: On the Origin,
    Management, and Prevention of Cancer.'
    https://youtu.be/VaVC3PAWqLk